HATHA YOGA
FOR ALL

Rajeswari Raman

MOTILAL BANARSIDASS PUBLISHERS
PRIVATE LIMITED • DELHI

First Edition: Bangalore, 1979
Second Edition: Delhi, 1991
Reprint: Delhi, 1993, 1995

ISBN: 81-208-0937-8

Also available at:

MOTILAL BANARSIDASS

41 U.A., Bungalow Road, Jawahar Nagar, Delhi 110 007
120 Royapettah High Road, Mylapore, Madras 600 004
16 St. Mark's Road, Bangalore 560 001
Ashok Rajpath, Patna 800 004
Chowk, Varanasi 221 001

PRINTED IN INDIA

BY JAINENDRA PRAKASH JAIN AT SHRI JAINENDRA PRESS,
A-45 NARAINA, PHASE I, NEW DELHI 110 028
AND PUBLISHED BY NARENDRA PRAKASH JAIN FOR
MOTILAL BANARSIDASS PUBLISHERS PRIVATE LIMITED,
BUNGALOW ROAD, DELHI 110 007

dedicated to my guru, friend, guide and husband dr. b. v. raman

A man should uplift himself by his own self, so let him ***not*** *weaken this self. For this self is the friend of oneself,* ***and*** *this self is the enemy of oneself.*

— **Srimad Bhagavad Gita**

CONTENTS

PREFACE TO THE SECOND EDITION

This Edition could not be brought out earlier for obvious reasons though there has been an ever-increasing demand for it.

I thank Motilal Banarsidass Publishers Pvt. Ltd., for bringing out the book in an attractive manner.

RAJESWARI RAMAN

PREFACE TO THE FIRST EDITION

The idea of writing a book on Yoga suitable to the average house-holder was prompted by my daughter Gayatri Devi Raman. I became interested when she started discussing the plans for this book. At first I was a bit hesitant, but as an avid follower of Yoga herself, my daughter won and I had to yield to her persuation.

In a book of this sort there are bound to be some repetitions and reiterations. But I feel that these enhance rather than detract from the value of the book.

I am thankful to my daughter Gayathri Devi Raman for her many excellent suggestions and her long hours of help during the writing of the book.

My thanks are also due to my sons B. Niranjan Babu and B. Sachidananda Babu for their assistance in proof-correction and to Messrs. P. N. Kamat and G. K. Anantaram of IBH Prakashana for bringing out this book so elegantly.

Bangalore **RAJESWARI RAMAN**
15-12-1978

INTRODUCTION

I have written this book so that more people will know about Yoga and what it is. Of course, there have been many books on the subject and mine is only just another. But I believe I can be an instrument in spreading the message of Yoga, in corners where it has not reached before. These corners are the lives of the middle-class women in our country whose sole activity is one of back-breaking chores. This section of women particularly requires the greatest attention since it is the pivot on which the entire household revolves morally, ethically and emotionally. Not that students or working girls do not need Yoga. They do. But they have better opportunity than the housewife chained to a life of constant work and responsibility. If she benefits from Yoga, the whole household will automatically but indirectly derive the benefit of a tranquil, smooth-run home.

Popularly believed to be exclusive to forest dwellers, this notion must be removed. Yoga is for everyone. No one is barred from its practice for reasons of sex, age or health or vocation. But there are some exceptions. Anyone can do it and emerge a more healthy and happier person than before. But Yoga, by its very nature, calls for patient and regular practice. It would certainly not be wise to expect results overnight like the wrinkled face that expects a flower-fresh complexion the next morning after using a beauty-cream. The cream may or may not give results even after regular application. But I can assure you, Yoga will. It does not cost anything. In fact, you save a lot on unnecessary items of expenditure when you begin to regulate your life through Yoga. All that Yoga requires is a corner of your house and a mat on which you can do the various asanas. And, half-an hour a day will save you endless visits to the doctor and medical bills for a life-time. This is certainly something worth trying in today's expensive world.

The break-neck pace of modern living with its attendant evils of restlessness, tension and nervous strain have cost us peace and tranquillity. It has given rise to new and unheard of health problems. Even our youth is falling prey to these problems and trying to escape from it all through pot, drugs and drink. Yoga, in this context, is a great boon. Many chain smokers and drug addicts have found their cravings disappear by the practice of Yoga which has given them a calm centre and a genuine sense of well-being.

I have limited myself to just the barest to give you an idea of Yoga in general and Hatha Yoga, in particular. I have not gone into the details for each bit of Yoga can very well fill hundreds of pages. No housewife in India would have the time for such volumes.

If by reading these pages, you find yourselves awakened to our great heritage of Yoga, my task in writing this book will have been sufficiently rewarded.

Bangalore
15-12-1978

RAJESWARI RAMAN.

THE AUTHOR

Mrs. Rajeswari Raman, wife of Dr. B. V. Raman, the famous exponent of astrology and Indian culture, is self-educated in the various aspects of Indian Culture. Her interest in Yoga started even as a young girl, her talents taking concrete shape as her children began to grow up.

By diligent study and practice she has mastered certain Yogic techniques and has been giving instruction to a number of ladies who seek her help to overcome their physical or mental ills. Letters of appreciation (some of which we reproduce in the latter part of the volume) are being received from different parts of the world from persons who have been benefited by her advice. She is not a professional, though.

Solely actuated by the desire that her sisters should share her experiences in the field of Yogic techniques so that they could preserve their mental and physical health and face the problems of life squarely, she started the Surya Prakash Institute of Yoga for Women in 1968 in memory of her eldest son Sri B. Surya

Prakash who passed away in 1963; it was Yoga that enabled her to stand this shock.

As the Director of the Institute Mrs. Raman is not only reassuring that women, given a chance, could muster sufficient courage to rely on themselves for their own emancipation from physical, mental and spiritual malaise, but more important also demonstrating that Indian women are essentially the repositories of India's rich and ancient culture which blend the physical, mental and spiritual factors into a purposeful whole.

Mrs. Rajeswari Raman has been delivering demonstration-talks to propagate Yoga and certain lasting values of life which are held dear from times immemorial in our country and culture.

During her world tour in 1970 with her husband Dr. Raman, Mrs. Rajeswari gave lectures in different parts of Europe and America and created in the minds of our Western sisters a keen interest in Yoga and the Hindu values of life.

She is of the view that the craze for the kind of happiness, outward happiness derived from external aids alone that has gripped the average man and woman should give place to the Indian view that the crux of one's happiness,

CHAPTER I

YOGA

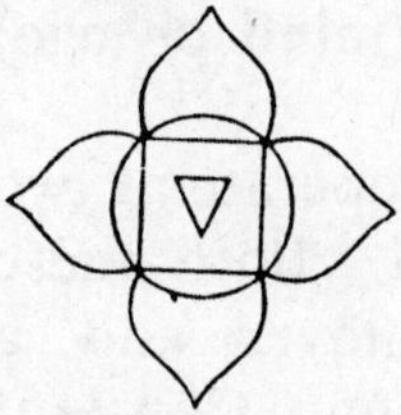

Health is the highest gain, contentment the greatest wealth. A trustworthy person is the best kinsman; Nirvana is the highest bliss.

– Dhammapada

The word Yoga automatically calls to mind Sage "Patanjali" the founder and father of Yoga. He lived around three centuries before Christ, and was a great philosopher and grammarian. He was also a physician and a medical work is attributed to him. However, this work is now lost in the pages of time.

His best known work is *Patanjali Yoga Sutras* or Aphorisms on Yoga. The path outlined is called Raja Yoga or the sovereign path. It is so called because of the regal, noble method by which the self is united with the Overself.

Patanjali's Yoga has essentially to do with the mind and its modifications. It deals with the training of the mind to achieve oneness with the Universe. Incidental to this objective are the acquisition of siddhis or powers.

The aim of Patanjali Yoga is to set man free from the cage of matter. Mind is the highest form of matter and man freed from this dragnet of Chitta or Ahankara (mind or ego) becomes a pure being.

The mind or Chitta is said to operate at two levels—intellectual and emotional. Both these levels of operation must be removed and a dispassionate outlook replace them. Constant Vichara (enquiry) and Viveka (discrimination between the pleasant and the good) are the two means to slay the ego enmeshed in the intellect and emotions. Vairagya or dispassion is said to free one from the pain of opposites—love and hate, pleasure and pain, honour and ignominy, happiness aud sorrow.

The easiest path to reach this state of dispassion and undisturbed tranquility is the path of Bhakti or love. Here, man surrenders his all—mind, soul, ego—to the Divine Being and is only led on by the Divine Will. Self-surrender must be cultivated through Japa or recitation of the Divine Name. Such repetition must not be mechanical but one-pointed and full of fervour.

For this, concentration is necessary. Concentration can be there only if man has practised to fix his attention on a particular object without letting it dwell on anything else.

Concentration also calls for regulation of conduct if Bhakti must develop. Good cheer, compassion, absence of jealousy, complacence towards the virtuous and consideration towards the wicked must be consciously cultivated.

There are also methods of regulated breathing which help reach concentration.

Yoga is an art and takes into purview the mind, the body and the soul of the man in its aim of reaching Divinity. The body must be purified and strengthened through various practices. The mind must be cleansed of all gross and the soul should turn inwards if a man should become a yogic adept. Study purifies the mind and surrender takes the soul towards God.

The human mind is subject to certain weaknesses which are universal. Avidya—wrong notions of the external world, asmita—wrong notions of oneself, raga—longing and attachment for sensory objects and affections, dwesha—dislike and hatred for objects and persons, and abinivesha or the love of life are the five defects of the mind that must be removed. Constant meditation and introspection eradicate these mental flaws.

The human body is a vehicle for journeying this life. It must be kept in proper form if the mind should function well. For this, there are practices too, but Patanjali does not elucidate on them.

The Yoga of Patanjali is Ashtanga or comprised of 8 limbs.
They are :

1. Yama
2. Niyama
3. Asana
4. Pranayama
5. Pratyahara
6. Dharana
7. Dhyana and
8. Samadhi.

Ahimsa (non-injury), satya (truth), asteya (non-covetousness), brahmacharya (continence) and aparagriha (abstinence from avarice) come under Yama.

These five austerities are universal and absolute. Under no condition should they be deviated from. A Yogi must not cause injury or pain to another in thought, word or deed. One must not hurt even in self-defence. This is Ahimsa.

Truth is concurrence between thought, word and deed. It must be true to fact and at the same time pleasant. If by speaking the truth, another is hurt it ceases to be truth and becomes himsa. There is a story which illustrates this point.

In olden days there was a sage renowned for his austerities and observance of the vow of truth. It so happened that once when he was sitting by his little hut, a frightened man with a bundle ran past him and disappeared into a cave nearby. A couple of minutes later there came a band of fierce robbers with gleaming knives, apparently looking for this man. Knowing that the sage would not lie, they asked him where the man with the bundle was hiding. At once, the sage, true to his vow of not uttering falsehood, showed them the cave. The cruel robbers rushed into it, dragged out the scared man, killed him mercilessly and departed with his bundle. The sage never realised God in spite of his austerities and tenacity for truth for he had been instrumental in the murder of a man. This is not the kind of truth that yoga requires. It would have been better if the sage had remained quiet for that would have saved the poor man. Great care is therefore to be exercised in speaking and each word must be carefully weighed before it is uttered.

There is a story in the *Chandogya Upanishad* which illustrates truth. It was the practice for little boys, in those days, to seek out a Guru for learning all about the Soul. Satyakama was one such little boy, eager to find a Guru who would teach him all that his young heart yearned for.

He went to his mother and said, "Mother, who is my father and what is my gotra (lineage)? I must tell my Guru all this before he will accept me as his student."

Satyakāma's mother was Jabala, who had worked as a servant in many households and who did not know the boy's father herself. But she knew how eager her little boy was to gain in knowledge and so, overcoming her own confusion, said : "My little boy, I worked in many houses as a maid and I conceived you. I do not know your father. But I can tell you I am Jabala and you are Satyakama."

Armed with this answer, the boy left his mother and went in search of a Guru. He came to Haridrumata Gautama, a renowned master. The first question the Guru asked was "Boy, tell me your lineage."

Straightaway the little boy answered with confidence, "I am Satyakama Jabala", and narrated all that his mother had told him.

The great Haridrumata was pleased with the truthfulness of the boy and at once accepted him as a student.

Hear, we notice the boy did not refrain from

speaking out the truth, although it could have denied him his most cherished object of learning. Only in this case the Guru was great enough to recognise the little boy's greatness and did not dismiss him away as a bastard.

What is Truth can never be defined but certain broad guidelines can be laid down.

"Truth is not the same as fact. It is an announcement of reality but subject to :—

"1. It is wrong to speak the truth when by doing so, one betrays another person unnecessarily and to no good purpose.

"2. Be protective about others' faults so long as they harm no one else. Speak privately to an offender about his failings—but only if you have an opportunity or responsibility to help him; but never, under the pretext of helping someone, speak deliberately to hurt him.

"3. Truth is always wholesome fact; a fact that can never be harmful. A fact which harms another, even if the truth must not be published or spoken. Never reveal unpleasant facts that cause meaningless suffering to another such as speaking out unnecessarily against another's character. Your hurtful action will not only cause pain, but rebound and do you also harm."

Non-covetousness is not hankering after things not one's own. Longing for things belonging to another breeds infatuation for the object and clouds thinking. It leads to theft and pilfering. No matter how insignificant the object, in principle, the mind is stained if once one begins to covet another's things.

Continence is abstinence from sexual intercourse. The abstinence must be complete. Although physically controlling oneself, if one mentally dwells on it, there is no real continence.

The vow of Brahmacharya is one of the hardest to keep up. It requires great vigil and watchfulness. Thoughts of lust are always lurking in the bottom of the mind and waiting to erupt. Even great sages have succumbed to temptation. Shakuntala was born to Menaka of of Viswamitra, a great tapaswin when he let himself be enamoured of the celestial dancer.

How insidiously lust takes possession of a person is shown in the following story.

Many students were learning Vedanta at the hermitage of a great master. After a discourse on Brahmacharya, the master added finally, "Beware, students. Always keep away from women. No matter how staunch your resolution and self-control, proximity leads to desire and desire, to ruin."

One of the students who thought very highly of himself interrupted : "No master, that cannot be. I am perfected in Brahmacharya and nothing can tempt me."

The master smiled to himself and dismissed the class. The students were sent to different parts of the country to preach to the people.

This student also left on his preaching mission and set himself up in a small hut in a village. One day, it began to rain heavily. He stood by the door of his hut watching the rain when a young girl, who was in the flush of her youth, came running to take shelter under a tree opposite the hut. The rain grew worse and it began to grow dark. The student felt sorry for the drenched girl, and invited her to come into the hut. She came. Soon it was night and the student gave the girl clothes to change and a mat to lie down on in the outer room. But his mind kept going back to the girl and suddenly he was driven by an irresistible urge to embrace her. He took her in his arms when whom should he see but his master instead caught in his arms.

The master said, "Are you still so sure of your self-control ?"

The student hung his head in shame.

Perfect Brahmacharya cannot be advocated for an average person. That is why, our ancients set up the institution of marriage where a man's basic tendencies and instincts are taken into account and regulated. Excesses can lead to ruin—physical and moral.

Absence of avarice is the absence of the desire to acquire, to possess and enjoy objects. It is undesirable because the acquisition and preservation of possessions may necessitate forbidden means and the breaking of the earlier mentioned austerities.

A classic illustration of covetousness and avarice is found in the story of a mighty king. Once while on a hunting expedition, he came by the ashrama of Vasishta and decided his men needed some rest. He went into the ashrama and after prostrating himself before the Maharishi sought his hospitability. The sage agreed and soon fed the king and his countless soldiers with the most dainty dishes. Afterwards they were led to mansions filled with every kind of luxury and entertainment so that they could rest their tired bodies. The king was amazed and began to wonder how a hermitage could arrange for all this royal treatment. He found the sage had a cow Kamadhenu which could yield anything he wished for. The king was filled with desire for such a wonderful cow and decided he should possess it. He fought the sage with his mighty army but Kamadhenu razed the whole battalion effortlessly. The king lost his entire army and became mad with misery and covetousness for the wish-fulfilling cow. This is the story of

Vishwamitra before he became a Rishi. Desire breeds misery and blinds one to everything.

The observances or Niyamas are five in number. They are :

1. Saucha (cleanliness)
2. Santosha (contentment)
3. Tapas (purificatory penance)
4. Swadhyaya (study of sacred books) and
5. Ishwarapranidhanani (total surrender to the Divine Being)

Saucha is the cleanliness of the body and mind. The body is kept clean externally by washing and scrubbing. Internally it is cleaned by various methods.

The aim of Saucha is to create an awareness of what the body is and that it contains but flesh, filth, blood, mucus and is not worthy of the attachment and love we bestow on it. A thorough cleaning of the various orifices creates disgust and removes our infatuation for the body.

A great Bhakta of the Lord once fell a victim to lust and began courting a beautiful dancer. He soon forgot God and all his thoughts remained absorbed in the dancer. He began to ply her with gifts and ornaments. One day he found there was nothing left in his house and so he went to his sister-in-law to see if she could give him something for the dancer. The sister-in-law was an enlightened and intelligent woman. She thanked God she was given an opportunity to teach her brother-in-law a lesson. She took out her best jewels and gave them to the distraught Bhakta on a condition.

She said, "When you go to the dancer, ask her to stand naked before you. You must go behind her and ask her to bend forward. She must take the jewels from you in this posture through between her legs."

The Bhakta went to the dancer in joy and bade her receive the jewels in accordance with his sister-in-law's directions. No sooner did the dancer bend forward, the Bhakta was struck aghast at the ugliness and loathsomeness of the human body for which he had given up his dearest Lord. He was struck with remorse and went away to seek the Lord with greater and renewed dispassion.

Contentment is the ability to remain happy with whatever one has and not hanker after what one does not have. Saint Thyagaraja, a great composer and devotee of Sri Rama, sings in one of his songs "Santhamu Leka, Saukhymu Ledu" which means without contentment there can be no happiness.

Tapas is penance. It is training the body and mind to endure, without complaining the pairs of opposites—pain and pleasure, hunger and thirst, heat and cold, and practise fasts, vows and resolutions.

Tapas is often mistaken for torturing the body and distorting it out of all shape. Almost all temples in India are beseiged by beggars and sadhus. These sadhus stand on their hands or heads and claim to be great souls. Some of them pass rods of metal through their cheeks or tongue and other parts of the body. Yet others lie on beds of nails or swallow live cinders. Whatever all this is, it definitely is not Tapas. It is desecrating the human body which is meant to be a temple for the Divine.

Lord Krishna in his famous *Bhagavad Gita* tells us what tapas is. There are three kinds of tapas or austerity: Tapas of the body, of speech and of mind.

Tapas of the body is worshipping the devas, the twice born or Brahmanas or pious people, teachers and the wise, purity, upright posture, continence and non-violence.

Credible people are sometimes carried away by the sensational feats of sadhus and mistake them for realised souls. Abuse of the body cannot be tapas.

Austerity of speech consists of speech that does not vex others, truth, pleasant talk which is beneficial and the study of sacred scriptures.

Serenity of mind, sympathy, silence,

self-control and integrity of motive are called austerity of the mind.

Study of the scriptures leads to divine contemplation. Actually a man is known by the company he keeps. These days, how can one make out whether a sanyasi is a genuine one or a fraud. So instead of seeking such company, books are more helpful and indirectly become our teachers. Constant study of good books leads to contemplation. Contemplation leads to meditation and Bhakti for God.

Total surrender to the Divine Will erases the ego and starts the process of the evolution of the soul.

There is a little story that teaches what total surrender is. Once Lord Vishnu and his consort, Lakshmi were relaxing in Vaikunta over a game of dice. Suddenly Lord Vishnu got up in haste when Lakshmi intercepted him and asked him for the reason.

The Lord replied, "My devotee is in danger of being assaulted by armed thieves. He is calling Me", and in a trice was gone. But the next instant, He was back. Lakshmi was bewildered.

"You are back so soon ?" she asked him.

"Yes", sighed the Lord, "My devotee called Me, but in the meanwhile he had picked up a large stone to throw at the thieves and defend himself. He had more faith in himself and in the stone than in Me. And so, I came back."

Total surrender is the realization of our littleness and insignificance before the Almighty. Draupadi's story is another illustration. So long as she clung to the garment with her hands depending upon them to save her modesty, Lord Krishna did not turn up. But the moment she threw up her hands in supplication letting go the garment, the Lord came to her rescue.

In fact, Patanjali holds that what all can be achieved by the practice of the different stages of Yoga can be attained singly through Iswara-pranidhanani or total surrender of the self to God.

Yoga asanas are the next stage. Ordinarily, the life of a yogi is outwardly shorn of all activity. The limbs are used only when necessary. This does not conduce to good health. Asanas or Yogic postures, therefore, become important. Asanas help maintain health and vitality in an otherwise sedentary life. They also give steadiness to the body, an important factor in future yogic practices.

The next step is Pranayama. Prana is the life-giving force circulating through the human body. Although prana is commonly interpreted as 'breath', it is something more vital in function and more subtle in operation than breath.

Pranayama regulates the flow of Prana which purifies the dross in the mind and body.

Pratyahara comes next. It is the disengaging of the senses from the sense-objects. By sustained practice, the senses are trained to cease to dwell on external objects and turn inwards.

Once the outgoing senses are taught to look inwards, Dharana or concentration becomes easy. The mind is steadied, the thought processes slow down and attention is fixed uninterrupted on a particular object. The object may be an image of God or the tip of the tongue or the space between the eyebrows or even an imaginary radiance in one's heart. Continued fixity of attention leads to Dhyana or meditation. Meditation is the continuous flow of a single thought from the person meditating to the object meditated upon. Effortless concentration is, in a sense, Dhyana.

The final stage is Samadhi or Beautitude. In this, the person meditating and the object of meditation become one. There is complete identification between the two.

Dharana, Dhyana and Samadhi are collectively called Samyama or the means of acquiring all knowledge beyond the senses.

Samyama must be employed to evolve from plane to plane of superconsciousness. Samyama is said to bring in its wake supernatural powers and memory of past births. However, it must not be wasted in the pursuit of selfish ends and pleasures. The ultimate goal of all Yoga is Kaivalya or Emancipation of the Soul.

Kaivalya is that state when man experiences and perceives his Divinity. Divinity means perfection. Once this state is attained, there are no desires—the harbingers of misery and pain. Man becomes God or Bliss. Nothing disturbs his tranquility and happiness. This is the aim of Yoga. Only if we stop to think, we realise every thought and act we think or perform is really an attempt to reach happiness. But we are always looking for it in the wrong things and places. We do not get it there and we suffer anger, disappointment, and frustration. Again and again we look for it in the wrong places like the moth that is drawn towards the flame and gets destroyed.

Yoga shows us all happiness is within ourselves and trying to quench desires is like pouring ghee on fire which only makes it blaze more instead of putting it out. So with desire. It is never satisfied. Yoga shows us that happiness for which we are eternally searching can be obtained through non-desire.

To achieve a state of non-desire, the mind must be trained to think clearly. A healthy mind requires a healthy body. This is where Hatha Yoga comes in.

CHAPTER II

HATHA YOGA

> *Mind is the seed, Hatha Yoga is the soil and complete desirelessness is the water. With these three, the Kalpa-vrikhsa which is the Unmaniavastha springs up immediately.*
>
> – **Hathayogapradipika**

Yoga, as we have already seen, is the process of attaining self-realisation. However, we are concerned solely with Hatha Yoga with its object of purifying the body.

Hatha is derived from Ha meaning the Sun and Ta meaning the Moon. Yoga is derived from the Sanskrit term 'Yug' which means "yoke" or 'unite'. The two terms together denote the unification of the Sun and the Moon or the union of the Prana and Apana Vayus. This is a physical process regulating the inflow of breath in the two nostrils. But we must always remember that the purpose of Yoga, of any kind, is the evolution of the soul.

The mind, the body and the soul are the 3 parts of a human being, each separate in its apparent working but affecting the other in its functioning. There can be no divorce of the one from the other, and every one part is dependent on the other two for the efficiency and proper functioning of their sum total, *viz.*, the human being.

Conscious effort at body and mind control leads to an evolution of the soul which may be quite imperceptible. It is this result towards which all yogic practices are aimed. Yogic practice necessarily implies regulation and restraint of the bodily organs and functions and of the mental faculties.

Hatha Yoga as known to us today is drawn mostly from *Gheranda Samhita* and *Hathayoga-pradipika*. These two works seem to be from the same source since many lines from each repeat in the other.

Hatha Yoga can be divided into 7 heads :

1. Bodily purification
2. Asanas
3. Mudras
4. Pratyahara
5. Pranayama

6. Dhyana
7. Samadhi

I shall deal only with Asanas and Pranayama and touch upon one or two Mudras. I shall stress upon their importance in maintaining good health.

There are numerous asanas, but only some of them are important.

Anyone above 14 years of age can do Yoga-sanas. Sick people may also do them. Pregnant women must discontinue the practice after the 3rd month. Women must refrain from practice during the 4 days of menstruation each month. People suffering from heart disease must be careful and take up yogic practices only under expert supervision. Generally too, these asanas are best learnt from an able and competent teacher.

Asanas are best performed in the morning on an empty stomach. Where time does not permit they can be done in the evening, but at least 3 hours should elapse after the last meal. Regular practice at the same place and time gives good results soon.

Diet must also be regulated. Vegetarians can carry on with their usual food but excessively spicy, oily and rich foods should be reduced gradually, and wherever possible eliminated. Meat, eggs, fish are to be avoided. So also hard drinks. Freshly cooked food, fresh vegetables, plenty of fruits and greens and milk are the best foods for practitioners of Yoga subject, of course, to one's resources. Canned, refined and processed foods are best avoided since they can cause faulty elimination.

In other ways too, general life should be regulated by spacing work, rest and relaxation according to one's circumstances and means. As Lord Krishna himself says, "To him who is temperate in eating and recreation, in his effort for work, and in sleep and wakefulness, Yoga becomes the destroyer of misery."

If Hatha Yoga is faithfully practised, benefits will start showing in the form of a youthful face and figure, graceful posture and carriage, clear complexion, improved blood circulation and all-round general health.

Here are some interesting lines reproduced from "Perspectives in Yoga", a collection of Seminar papers edited by Dr A. K. Sinha.

"Prophylactic and Therapeutic Effects of Yogic Exercises.

"Academy of Research in Physical Culture, Warsaw, conducted studies on physiological and psychological aspects of Yoga system of exercise engaging the services of Romanowaski, Pasek and others to see if these could counteract the noxious effects of the contemporary environment on the ontogenesis of man (36, 42-48).

"Their results show that the ailments of the patients of Psychosomatic disorders of circulatory and digestive systems disapproved while their general considerable nervousness alleviated relatively slow pulse rate of 56-62 mim. And low arterial pressure 104-63-120/72 mim. Hg. were also noted. The examination of basal metabolism showed very low values of ventilation-4, 76% mint. on the average. The respiratory rhythm amounted to 4, 2/1/mim. the oxygen: consumption to 1/mim. of the air inhaled, *i.e.*, 20% greater than normal. The R.Q. in all the investigated in the resting position have been very low 0, 5-0, 7. This fact showed that the Oxygen utilisation by the tissues was larger than the average. Corresponding elimination of CO_2 had been increased. The EEG investigations indicated improved state of calmness in comparison to the control group with obvious symptoms of fatigue. Rorschach method proved that the experimental group represented the well balanced type of normal emotional reactivity as compared with their rather intensive neurotic background.

Hypertension:

"Datey and others studied 86 subjects (68 males and 18 females) of ages between 20 to 64 years. Their systolic blood pressure ranged between 160-270 and diastolic between 90-120 mm. H. There were 62 cases with essential, 19 with renal and 5 with arterio-sclerotic hypertension. They divided the whole population into 3 categories of (i) who had never received antihypertension drug, (ii) adequately controlled with drugs, (iii) inadequately controlled with drugs. In addition to blood pressure pulse rate, respiration, common symptoms were recorded and electromyographs were taken before and periodically during the study and after practice.

"With the practice of merely Shavasana, significant response was seen in about 60% of the patients despite the facts that some failures were due to irregularity in exercise and incorrect technique. The reduction in the mean Bp by 30 mm. Hg. symptomatic relief and increase in sense of well-being in most of the cases was seen. Electromyogram from frontalis and physiogram also showed improvement.

"A group of hundred patients showing symptoms of psychoneurosis and psychosomatic disorders including cases of anxiety, anxiety depression, hysteria etc., and comprising of 66 males and 34 females whose ages ranged from 16 to 64 years was taken for pilot study for the treatment by a therapeutic technique based upon some concepts of Patanjali by

Dr. Vahia and his co-workers of the Psychiatric Department at K.E.H. Hospital, Bombay. After the practice of two months duration the improvement in the condition of the patients was judged by opinions of the patients, relatives and the team of doctors engaged in the project. It was observed that the improvement rate was statistically significant........

"Kaivalyadhama S.M.Y.M. Samiti, Lonavla, financially helped by the Central and Maharashtra Governments undertook a project in 1964-65 to assess the value of yogic treatment in bronchial asthma patients numbering 139 were admitted in batches of eight for a period of four weeks each....Yogic treatment of asthma was helpful even in cases where all other known methods had failed (7).

"In his recent article on prevention and treatment of cancer by Yoga, Dr. Karambelkar, an eminent biochemist of Kaivalyadhama, Yoga Institute, quoting Dr. Poret's view that aeriological factors of cancer were phychological, psychical and spiritual on the basis of the findings of Prof. Vincene who found that the PH_1, RH_2 and RO of the venous blood of patients of cancer and neurosis fell into the same zone, believes that it is reversible where alkaline PH and oxydation rH2 were below certain degree and successfully preventable by yogic exercises........

"The results of these investigations lead us to the conclusion that the judicious and progressive follow-up of yogic practices brings about higher and higher conditioning of limbic system which is thought to be responsible for regulation of ANS, endocrinal system and the affective behaviour. It appears that the practitioners gradually begin experiencing greater and greater volitional control over the metabolic and the autonomic functions of the body which leads to the recovery of homeostatic dysfunction in the case of the sick and towards perfection of biological equilibrium in the case of normal persons. How such changes are brought about is still not so very clear andrequires further investigations regarding the mechanism through which yogic exercises produce physiological and mental effects."

Many people somehow have the notion that if they stop practising Yoga, they put on weight. Frankly, I should like to point out this is an unfair charge. The very reason they start on the Yoga course is their overweight problem. As they continue the practice, they find they are reducing. At once they stop further practice and naturally, glandular irregularities (which are the ultimate reason for all overweight problems) which had been under regulation through Yoga, start all over again. In such cases, my honest answer would be to ask them if their own laziness to do the Yoga exercises is not responsible for such a situation. They forget the fact, and ungratefully too, that the fat they had accumulated in their bodies for years through indiscriminate eating and laziness had been fast disappearing through Yoga. Instead of blaming themselves for lazily giving up Yoga, they shift the blame on this ancient art. Show me just one person who has put on weight after giving up Yoga, but who was not fat before. You just will not come across any such case. I have noticed over many years people will talk about beauty, health, and trim figures day and night, and pore over magazines and books for tips but will do nothing about it. They are too lazy and so much in love with themselves they will not admit it but prefer to throw the blame on Yoga. The very fact Yoga has survived such slandering over the centuries is sufficient defence and proof of the amazing results it can give.

CHAPTER III

MEDITATIVE POSES

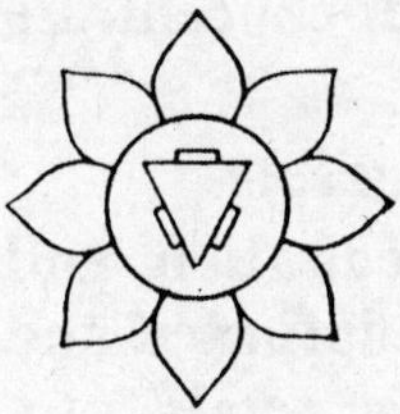

When the breath wanders, the mind is steady, but when the breath is still, so is the mind.

– **Hathayogapradipika**

These poses are so designed by the ancient sages who discovered them, that they enable one to sit in the same pose for hours together at a stretch steadily and without jerks. This steady posture enables one to attain one-pointedness of mind.

Padmasana is the famous lotus-pose commonly known as the Buddha pose. Siddhasana is another pose generally used for meditation.

Practise each pose starting with a few seconds in the beginning and gardually increase the period to 15 minutes and more. Three hours is the maximum period allowed for a layman, but you can sit in the asana for this period only after years of practice.

In all these meditative poses, sit erect with the head, neck and trunk in one straight line. After assuming the pose gaze steadily at any fixed object without letting your eyes dart about restlessly. Or else, close them and concentrate on your breath.

Padmasana (Lotus pose)

This is the best pose for meditation and japa. The soles of the two feet upturned and resting on the thighs resemble the petals of a lotus and hence, the name.

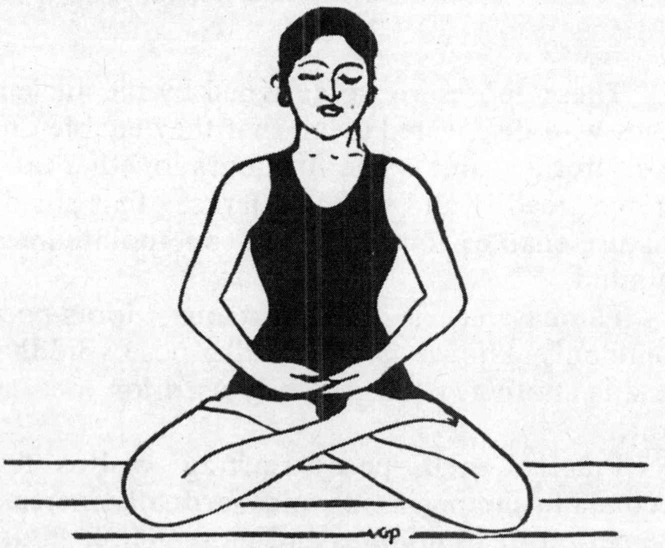

Padmasana

(1) Spread a blanket or carpet on the floor. If available, a deer skin can also be used and is always highly recommended if it is for dhyana or japa.

(2) Sit erect on it with the two legs outstretched.

(3) Take hold of the right foot and bending it at the knee, place it high on the left thigh, the sole upturned.

(4) Now, catch the left foot and place it symmetrically across the right ankle so that the foot rests on the right thigh.

(5) Adjust the feet high up against the thigh so that the upturned heels are as near the abdomen as possible.

(6) Place the palms one on top of the other over the upturned soles.

(7) Make sure the head, the neck and the trunk are in one straight line and the back is straight.

(8) Also make sure both the thighs and knees are pressed against the floor. You will find in the beginning one of the thighs slightly off the ground. Slowly and carefully press the thigh against the ground and retain the pose for a few seconds.

Benefits : Padmasana is an excellent posture for all meditative and pranayamic practices. It loosens the joints in the lower parts of the body and removes rheumatism. It tones up the three humours (wind, phlegm and bile) in the system harmonising their functions. It strengthens the nerves and muscles of the legs and thighs.

If you are used to eating on the floor as we do in India, Padmasana will be easy to assume. Otherwise, do not force yourself as this can injure you. By gradual practice, train the legs to assume the pose. However, three months should be enough even for one with very stiff legs to assume Padmasana properly.

Siddhasana (Pose of the Adept)

Siddha means an adept. Siddhasana is the pose of an adept.

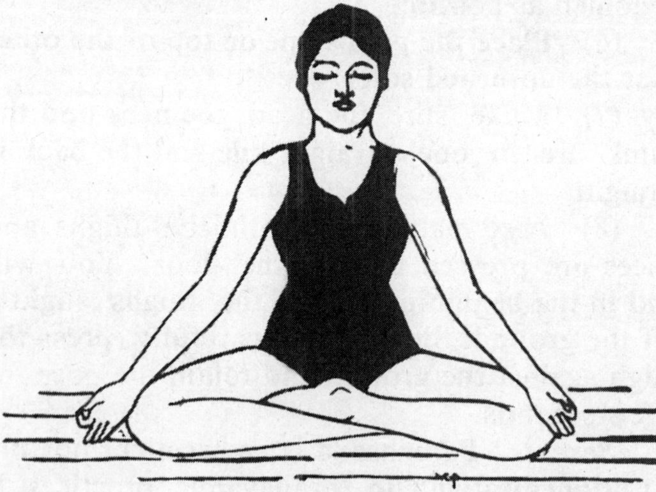

Siddhasana

1. Sit erect on the carpet with the legs outstretched as in the previous pose.

2. Take hold of the left foot, bend it at the knee and place the heel such that it presses against the anal aperture.

3. Next, bending the right foot also at the knee, place the right heel against the root of the reproductive organ taking care to see no pressure is felt on the delicate organs.

4. Place the hands with the palms one on top of the other on the feet as in Padmasana.

5. Make sure the head, neck and trunk are in one straight line.

Benefits : Siddhasana is also one of the best postures for meditation and concentration. It is supposed to help one get established in Brahmacharya or celibacy.

Siddhasana is easier to assume than Padmasana. Novices can practise this first before attempting Padmasana particularly if they are not used to squatting on the floor.

CHAPTER IV

THE ASANAS

To him who is temperate in eating and recreation, in his effort for work, and in sleep and wakefulness, Yoga becomes the destroyer of misery.

– Srimad Bhagavad Gita

The asanas are poses mainly for health and strength. There are innumerable asanas, but not all of them are really necessary. I shall deal with only such asanas as are useful in curing ailments and maintaining good health. Asanas must be learned from a competent Guru or teacher who can make such changes or modifications in them as to suit the specific needs of a particular person. I shall outline very generally the method of some of these popular asanas. Breathing is very important in any asana and what I suggest is the simplest form of breathing.

The following points are important while practising Yoga :

(1) Always do asanas in a well-lit, clean and ventilated room. If you are one of those lucky few who can do it in the open in the privacy of your compound or terrace, so much the better. As far as possible, close the door of your room so that you are left undisturbed by people walking in and out of it.

(2) Wear minimum clothing, preferably cotton so that it does not interfere with breathing and perspiration. Discard all tight-fitting under-garments like corsets, belts and brassiers. Remove all footwear.

(3) Do the asanas on a blanket folded twice spread over a carpet. Use a bed-sheet over the blanket so that the woollen fibres do not stick to your lips or nose when you have to do the asanas that require you to lie on your stomach. It should not be too soft nor too hard.

(4) Tie your hair simply. Remove all pins and broaches and if you wear a bun, make sure it does not protrude unduly as to come in the way of your lying flat on the carpet.

(5) Always perform asanas early in the morning. If this is not possible, the next best time would be evening around dusk.

(6) Never do asanas on a full stomach immediately after a meal. Make sure at least 5 hours have elapsed after a heavy meal and at least 3 hours after a light meal (tiffin). You must allow at least half-an-hour to pass after a drink—tea, coffee, milk, juice, etc.

(7) Always seek the guidance of a competent teacher.

You may wonder why in spite of repeatedly pointing out the absolute need for a Guru, I have explained the general techniques of asanas. It is because if by reading about them, an interest is kindled in you to pursue this wonderful subject seriously, my aim in writing these pages will have been fulfilled to a large extent. Once the wish to study Yoga is earnest and sincere, a true Guru will appear sooner or later.

Bhujangasana (Snake pose)

The asana derives its name because it resembles a snake with its hood raised. The head and chest raised represent the hood while the rest of the body lying flat, the body of the snake.

1. Lie down on the carpet on your stomach, face down.

2. Relax all your muscles.

3. Place the palms of the hand on the floor in line with the shoulders, each palm facing

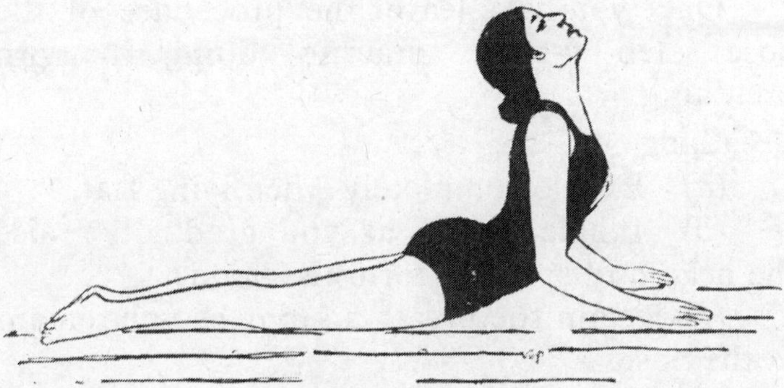

Bhujangasana

down and about 1 inch away from the tip of the shoulder.

4. Keep your feet together with the toes touching the ground.

5. Now slowly raise the head off the ground and take it up gradually so that the spine curves beautifully backwards. Do not exert force or do it suddenly. Each movement should be slow, continuous and without jerks.

6. Raise the spine little by little so that each vertebrae is gradually loosened.

7. Keep the body from the navel downwards touching the ground.

8. Retain the pose for a few seconds.

9. Gradually bring down the back to the original position of lying flat on your stomach.

10. Repeat the asana 6 times.

Once you have learnt the procedure of the pose step-by-step, practise doing it with breathing.

Breathing :

(*a*) Exhale completely when lying flat.

(*b*) Inhale slowly as you gradually raise the head and spine to form the hood.

(*c*) Retain the breath so long as you remain in the pose.

(*d*) Exhale slowly as you come down to your original position.

Benefits: Bhujangasana is one of the best asanas for all spinal and back-ache problems. The health and youth of a person depend upon the elasticity and suppleness of his back-bone. Most of us have noticed how as old age sets in, the back begins to stiffen. Bhujangasana tones up the entire spinal column pulling at the same time, the abdominal muscles. The pressure on these muscles gives relief from constipation. This asana is of particular help in toning up sluggish uterine muscles and ovaries. It is a powerful antidote against wet-dreams and leucorrhoea. It develops the chest and firms the bust.

Salabhasana (Locust pose)

This asana when fully assumed resembles a locust from which it derives its name.

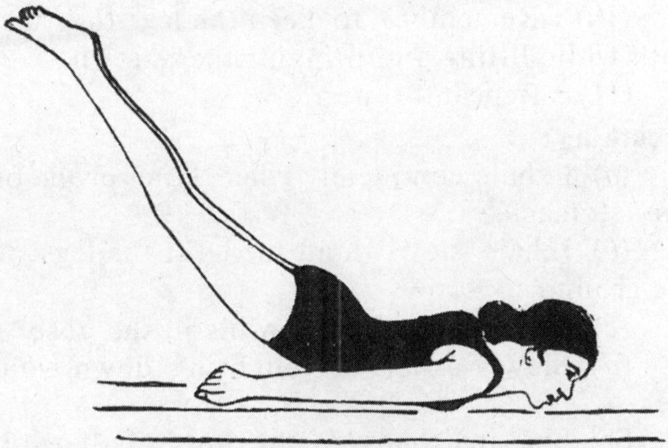

Salabhasana

(1) Lie flat on your stomach.

(2) Let the hands relax alongside the body, the palms facing upwards.

(3) Press the nose, forehead and chin against the ground.

(4) First let the whole body relax.

(5) Next stiffen all the muscles and raise the legs off the ground.

(6) Lift it as high as possible. Do not force it the first time but do it in measures by gradual practice.

(7) Do not bend the legs at the knees, but hold them from the thighs to the toes in a straight line.

(8) Retain the pose for a few seconds.

(9) Slowly bring the feet down.

(10) Remember to keep the legs together, both while lifting and bringing them down.

(11) Repeat 4 times.

Breathing:

(*a*) Exhale completely when lying prone on your stomach.

(*b*) Inhale slowly and then lift the legs off the ground.

(*c*) Retain your breath while in the pose.

(*d*) Slowly exhale as you bring down your feet.

Salabhasana tones up the lower half while Bhujangasana exercises the upper half of the body.

Benefits: This asana tones up the liver, kidneys and pancreas strengthening the muscles in these regions. The pressure against th abdomen stimulates the intestines removing sluggishness of the bowels. It tones up the vertebral column supplying plenty of blood to this region. It strengthens the pelvis and tones up the uterus. It rids one of flatulence.

Dhanurasana (Bow pose)

The body in this pose has the appearance of a bow with the string taut.

1. Lie flat on your stomach on a carpet.
2. Relax the entire body.

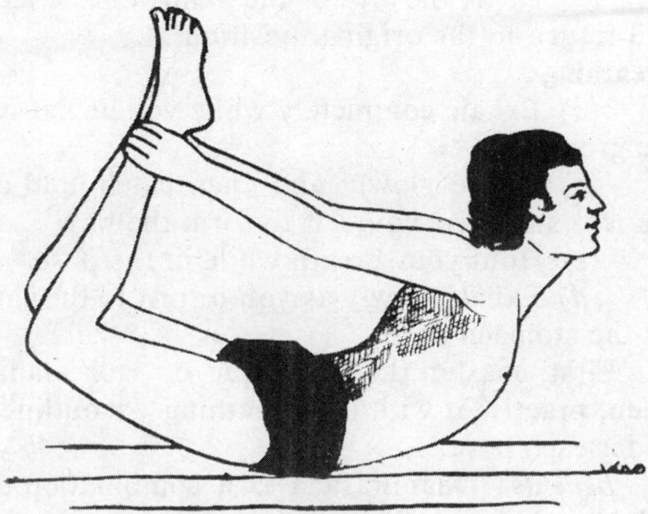

Dhanurasana

3. Bend the legs backward over the thighs.

4. Catch hold of each leg at the ankle with the hand.

5. Now, slowly raise the head and chest off the ground.

6. Next, raise the legs at the thighs higher and higher without undue force.

7. Tug at the legs with hands until the back arches beautifully while the hands hold the legs tight like the string of a bow.

8. Retain the pose for a few seconds balancing only on the abdominal region without any jerks or shakiness.

9. Relax the grip of the hands on the legs and return to the original position.

Breathing :

(*a*) Exhale completely while you lie flat on the ground.

(*b*) Inhale slowly and then catch hold of the legs and raise yourself to form the bow.

(*c*) Hold your breath while in the pose.

(*d*) Exhale slowly as you return to the flat-on-the-stomach pose.

First, master the technique of each asana. Then, practise it with the breathing as outlined under each pose.

Benefits: Dhanurasana is a combination of Salabhasana and Bhujangasana and gives the benefits of both. The entire back is massaged. It reduces obesity, cures constipation and rheumatism. It removes intra-uterine troubles, regulates menstruation and reduces greatly pains in the pelvic region. The practice of these three asanas regularly can be very useful in making labour and delivery smooth and almost painless.

Paschimottanasana

1. Lie flat on your back on the carpet.
2. Make sure the knees are also flat and pressed to the ground. Let the hands lie alongside the body.
3. Relax the body completely.

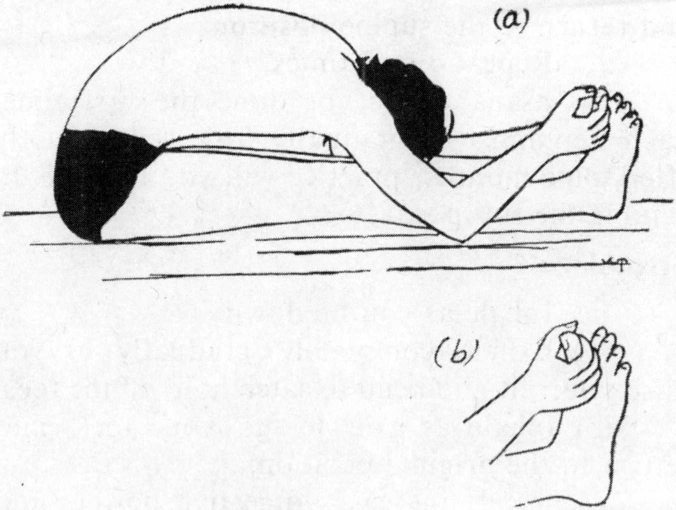

Paschimottanasana

4. Now, slowly lift yourself to a sitting position.

5. Bend forward and clasp the big toe of each foot with your index and middle finger Fig (*b*). There should be absolutely no strain or undue force.

6. Bring down your head so that it touches the knees. Do not raise your knees to achieve this, but let them remain fixed to the ground and straight Fig (*a*).

7. Remain in this pose for about 5 seconds.

8. Gradually release your grip on the toes and return to the supine position.

9. Repeat 4 or 5 times.

This asana cannot be done the first time. Each step must be gradually followed and only after some months' practice will you be able to assume the full pose.

Breathing :

(*a*) Inhale as you lie down.

(*b*) Exhale completely gradually as you raise yourself and bend to catch hold off the toes.

(*c*) Inhale as you let go your toes and return to the original position.

Benefits: It increases digestive powers and removes loss of appetite. The kidneys, liver, pancreas and abdominal muscles are stimulated. It gives relief from piles and diabetes. The legs are stretched to their fullest toning up the ham-string muscles. The spine is also massaged thoroughly. It is a good antidote for back-ache.

Halasana (Plough pose)

This is for all practical purposes the reverse of Paschimottanasana.

1. Lie flat on the carpet with the hands limp alongside.

2. Press the hands down on the ground as you lift the legs off the carpet.

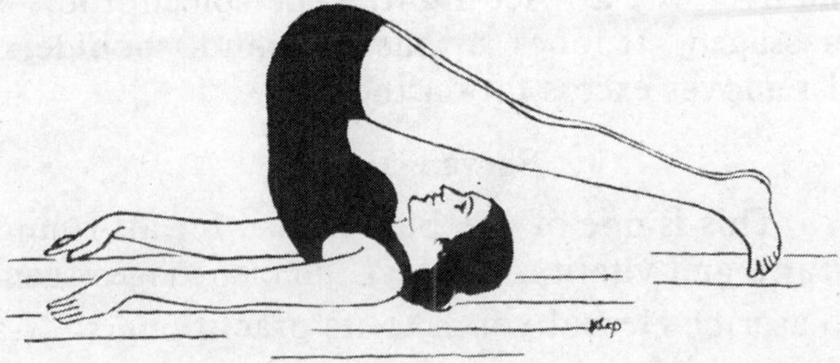

Halasana

3. Without bending at the knees, raise the hips higher and bring the legs over the head and backwards till the toes touch the ground.

4. Keep the knees straight and the legs together in a straight line.

5. Remain in the pose for a few seconds, and return to your original position.

6. Repeat 4 to 5 times.

Breathing :

Breathe slowly through the nose when in the pose. At other times, just breathe normally.

Benefits : In this asana, the muscles of the back are stretched fully and then relaxed. Every part of the vertebral column receives a rich supply of blood. Most ailments are caused by the poor condition of the spine. Halasana is an excellent tonic for maintainingthe spine in its best condition. It makes the posterior region elastic. Constipation and sluggish working of the liver are all set right. The spleen too, is massaged. It tones up the neck and shoulders. It removes excess fat on the hips.

Sarvangasana

This is one of the best asanas for all-round health and vitality. In fact, ancient sages seem to ascribe eternal youth to its practitioners. As

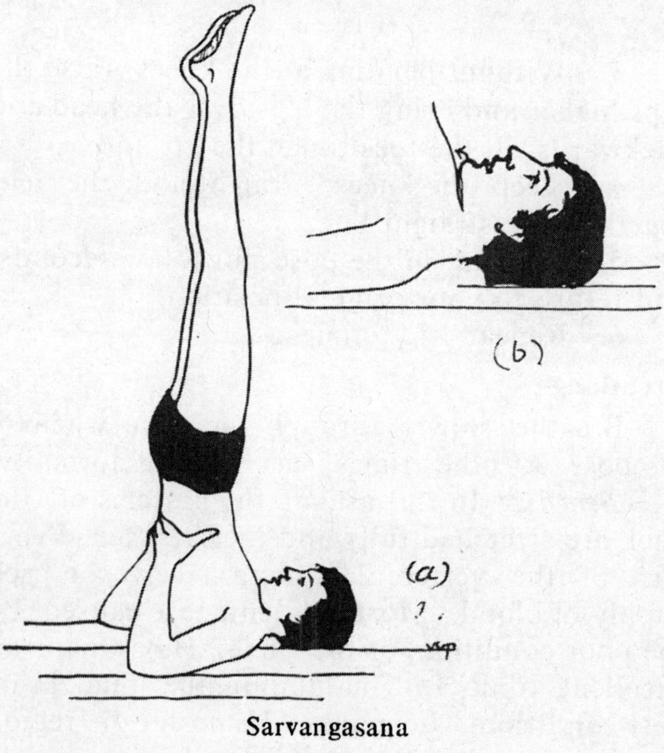

Sarvangasana

its very name suggests, it tones up all the organs (sarva-anga) of the system.

1. Lie down on a carpet with the hands by your side.

2. Slowly lift your legs off the ground, then the thighs and lastly, the hips.

3. Support the whole body—back, hips, thighs and legs—on your elbows, the hands pressing against the sides of the back for support.

4. Try to keep it as vertical as possible.

5. You will now find the chin pressing against the chest Fig. (*b*).

6. The shoulders, the neck and part of the head should touch the ground when the asana is properly done.

7. Keep the body steady without shaking or jerking the legs.

8. Remain in the asana for a few seconds and train to retain the pose for a maximum period of five minutes Fig. (*a*).

9. Gradually bring down the whole body and return to the original supine position.

This asana may be done just once.

Breathing :

Breathe slowly when in the pose.

Benefits : This asana, like the famous Sirshasana, reverses the whole body below the neck. The rich supply of blood to the face and the neck acts as a beauty treatment banishing unwelcome signs of age, wrinkles and grey hair. The chin-lock exerts pressure on the thyroid gland, toning it up. Ugly lines on the neck disappear. Double chins melt away. The blood from the legs flows down so that varicose veins are also cured. It also cures piles, constipation, poor blood circulation, female disorders and nocturnal emission. It keeps the urinary organs in good shape. It prevents premature hardening of the bones or ossification. It is even believed to cure leprosy.

In fact, this asana is believed to "destroy decay and death". Many beautiful women—models, filmstars and actresses—do this asana regularly to keep away the ravages of time. The enormous supply of blood to the head gives sparkling eyes. This asana is a good tonic for over-worked brains.

Caution : Do not attempt this asana if you are a heart patient or suffer from blood pressure, sinus trouble and weak eyes.

Matsyasana (Fish pose)

Sarvangasana must always be followed by Matsyasana. The former exerts a gentle pressure on the thyroid while the latter stretches the area containing the glands acting in just the opposite way on them.

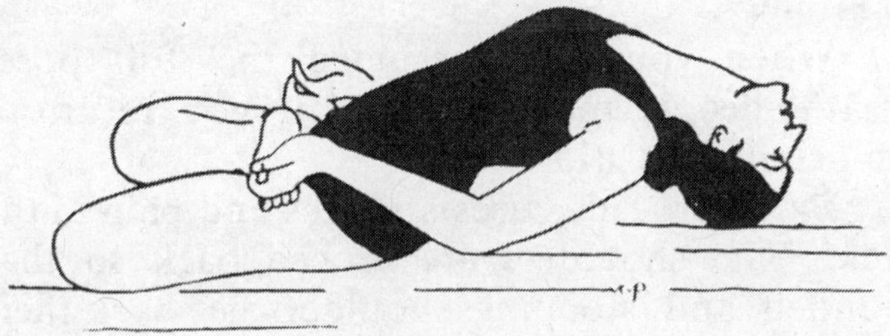

Matsyasana

1. Sit on a carpet and assume Padmasana.

2. Gently bring the body backwards down so that now you lie on the carpet but with the legs in Padmasana.

3. Let the elbows remain on the ground.

4. Lift the back off the ground, so that only the legs and head touch the ground, while the hands are also on the ground.

5. Throw the head well back so that the neck and back arch up and the body rests on the legs (in Padmasana) and the back of the head.

6. Catch hold of the toes with your hands, all the time the elbows touching the ground.

7. Remain in this pose for a few seconds and with practice learn to stay in it for 2 to 3 minutes.

8. Gently let go the toes, bring the back down and unclasp your legs from Padmasana.

You need not repeat this asana either.

Breathing :

When you have assumed the full pose, breathe deeply and slowly until you return to the original position.

Benefits: This cures stiffness and pain in the neck. The shoulders are arched back so that rounded and stooping shoulders get back their natural shape. The stretching of the trunk, waist and neck strengthens them and removes extra fat from these areas. The ribcage and lungs expand so that they are toned up and get fresh air and a bountiful supply of oxygen. Disorders of the pituitary and pineal gland are set right.

Mayurasana (Peacock pose)

1. Kneel down on the carpet.
2. Rest the palms on it facing downwards. Fig. (*c*)
3. Keep the hands firm and bring down the abdomen so that it presses against the elbows Fig. (*a*).
4. Stretch your legs back.
5. Now, raise them off the ground balancing at your abdomen on the support formed by the elbows Fig. (*b*).
6. Retain the pose for a few seconds steadily without tossing or shaking.
7. Return to the original pose.

This asana is not so easy it seems. Learning to balance will take at least three months while training to retain it without jerks, another three months.

Breathing :

(*a*) Inhale as you raise the legs off the ground.

(*b*) Retain the breath while in the pose.

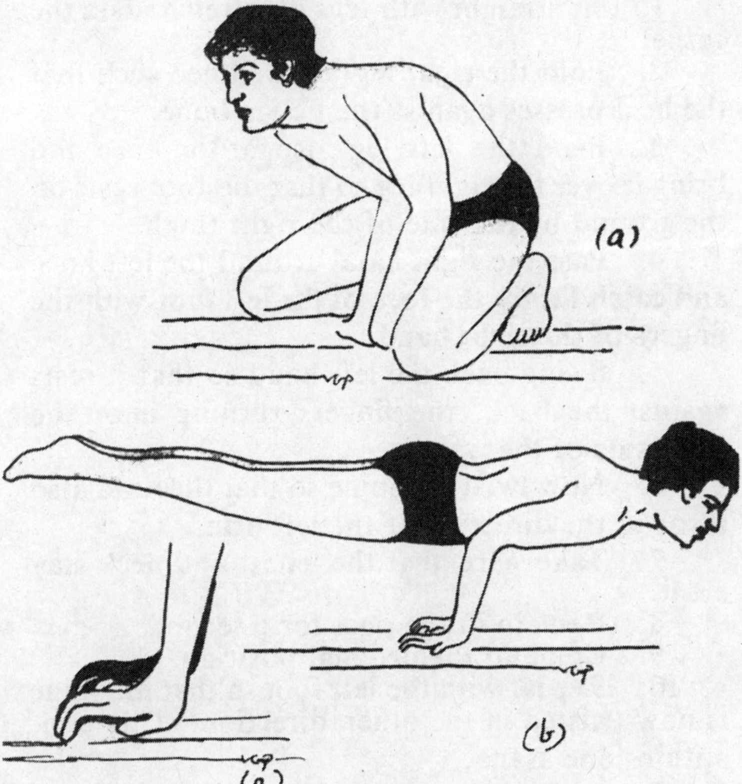

Mayurasana

(*c*) Slowly exhale while releasing the pose.

Benefits: This cures all types of stomach disorders. The liver, spleen and other digestive organs are toned up leading to better digestion and assimilation of food. It steadies mental tossing also.

Ardha-Matsyendrasana

1. Sit straight with legs outstretched on the carpet.
2. Fold the right leg at the knee such that the heel presses against the pelvic bone.
3. Bend the left leg also at the knee and bring it over the right leg so that the foot rests on the ground by the side of the right thigh.
4. Pass the right hand around the left knee and catch firmly the toes of the left foot with the fingers of the right hand.
5. Swing back the left hand so that it rests against the back, the fingers turning in on the right side of the waist.
6. Now twist the spine so that the head also turns in the direction of the left arm.
7. Take care that the chest and neck stay erect.
8. Remain in the pose for 5 seconds.
9. Come to the original position.
10. Repeat with the left foot so that the spine is now twisted in the other direction. This constitutes one asana.

Repeat 2 times.

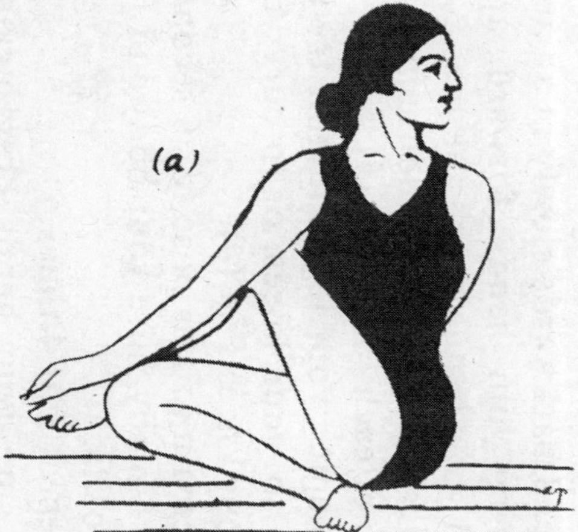

Ardha-Matsyendrasan

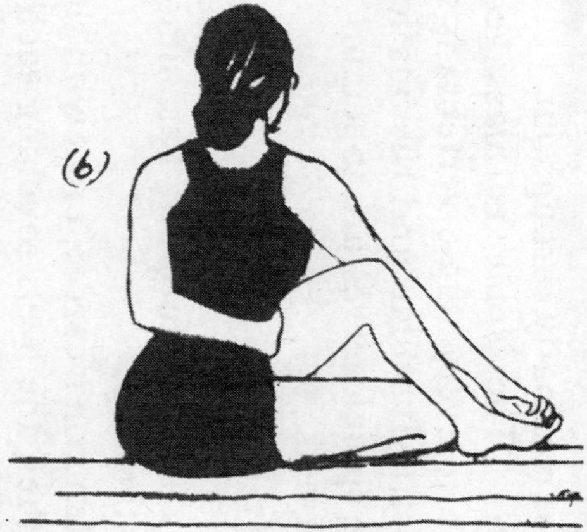

Ardha-Matsyendrasana

Breathing :

Breathe normally throughout.

Benefits: The spine is massaged in both directions and every single vertebra is stimulated by the twist. Muscular and rheumatic pains are cured. The spinal nerves are toned up. The waist line is trimmed.

Padahastasana

This is another form of Paschimottanasana but done standing.

1. Stand on a carpet, erect with the two feet close together, the heels touching each other.
2. Lift your hands high over the head.
3. Bend backwards slowly in an arch.
4. Bring your hands forward and bend down until your hands touch the toes.
5. Clasp the index and middle fingers round the big toe of each foot Fig. (*b*).
6. Keeping your legs straight, try to touch your nose to your knees or to bury your head between your knees Fig. (*a*).
7. Remain in this pose for 6 seconds.
8. Gradually raise your body and return to standing position.
9. Repeat 3 or 4 times.

Make sure your hands press against your ears throughout all the movements. This pose

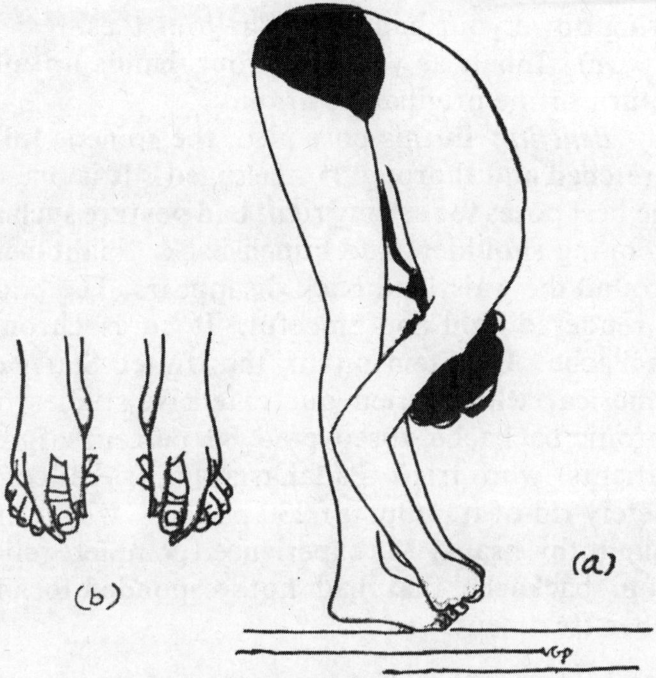

Padahastasana

requires long practice before it can be assumed fully. You should not force yourself to do it the first time. Even touching the toes with legs straight may not be possible at first. But by steady practice, you will be able to do it well soon.

Breathing :

(*a*) After you raise your hands above your head, inhale deeply as you arch your back backwards.

(*b*) Exhale slowly as you bend forward and bring down your hands to grip your toes.

(*c*) Inhale as you raise your hands up and return to the original position.

Benefits: In this pose also, the spine is fully stretched and thoroughly massaged. It is one of the best poses for setting right bad posture such as stooping shoulders and hunch-back. Flabbiness around the waist and back disappears. The body is rendered light and graceful. It cures chronic backache. Dr. Stemson of the United States of America, who carried out extensive studies on chronic backache, discovered 80 percent of the patients who tried Padahastasana were completely rid of it. Out of 230 patients who were taught this asana, 185 experienced complete relief from backache that had not responded to any other treatment.

Savasana

Now we come to the most important and unquestionably the most difficult asana. It is called the corpse-pose because it resembles one.

1. Lie flat on your back.

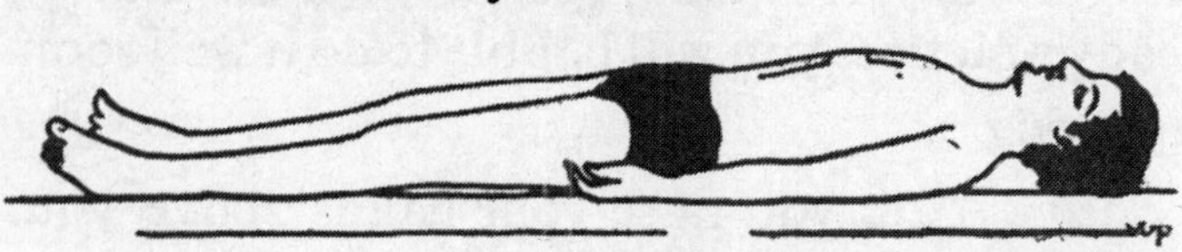

Savasana

2. Let the hands rest alongside.

3. Keep the legs straight and together with the heels touching.

4. Relax all the muscles in the body. Start with the toes and feel they are becoming limp and leaden. Next the ankles, the calves, the thighs, the hips, the abdomen, the heart, the shoulders, the neck, the arms, the elbows, the palms, every single finger and finally the head, the eyes, the lips, the ears and every single part of you.

5. By the time you do this, a feeling of great repose and relaxation will overtake you.

6. You will find your breathing will have slowed down and become more regular and fine.

7. Remain in this pose for 5 minutes to begin with and increase to 20 minutes.

8. Turn to your left, count 12, then turn to your right, count 12 and then get up on your right side.

At first you may find your different organs disobeying you and automatically fidgetting and restless. This is because you have never tried to consciously relax them. But with practice you will be able to still them.

This asana is excellent for anger, irritation, blood pressure and all those modern-day ailments that are the result of today's fast-paced life. In fact, many heart specialists prescribe regular practice of Savasana for sick hearts. Hypertension and blood-pressure patients benefit greatly by the practice of Savasana.

Sirashasana

The word Yoga to many people is still synonymous with Sirashasana, the topsy-turvy pose. Rightly too, for, this asana gives the maximum physical and spiritual benefits.

1. Spread a soft blanket on the floor.
2. Sit on your knees and bend down so that the crown of the head is on the blanket.
3. Interlock your fingers and place them on the blanket in such a way that the locked fingers form a support around the crown of the head. Rest the elbows on the ground forming a 'V' with the interlocked fingers as the vertex Fig (*d*).
4. Make sure your head is resting on the crown of the skull and not on the forehead.
5. Bring the knees close to the head with the toes pressing on the ground.
6. Remove the toes from the ground and throw up your legs. Fig (*a*).
7. Slowly raise them high until they are vertical and the whole body from the head up is in one straight line. Make sure the spine does not curve but remains straight Fig. (*b*) & (*c*).
8. Remain in this pose for a few seconds breathing slowly.

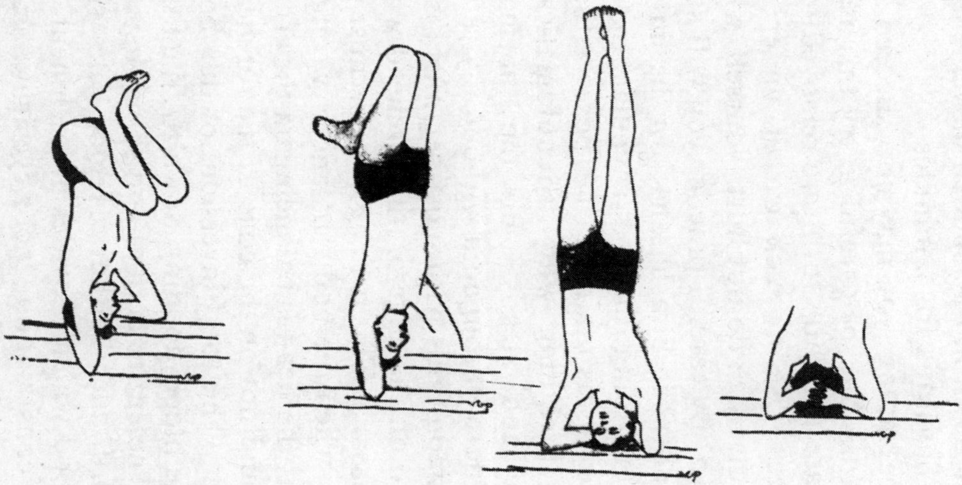

(*a*) (*b*) (*c*) (*d*)

Sirshasana

9. Bring the legs down gradually in stages. Do not come down in one sudden movement.

10. Do Savasana for 2 minutes.

In the beginning you may not succeed and may fall down. So, be careful to try this asana in a free space with all furniture removed to a safe distance. Use a thick carpet under the blanket so that you do not hurt yourself when you fall down. By careful practice you will soon become an adept in Sirashasana. In the initial stages, the breathing may be irregular but as you advance in maintaining the pose without jerks, your breathing will also automatically become fine and steady. Breathe normally through the nose throughout without any retention. A common fault with most beginners is to rest the head on the edge of the forehead while doing Sirashasana. This is dangerous because the spine curves when the body balances wrongly. So check that the head is balancing on the crown of the skull and not on the edge of the forehead.

Benefits : The total inversion of the body results in the blood flooding down to the heart and brain. The entire cranial and spinal nerves, the spinal cord, and the thorax region get a rich supply of blood which provides nourishment. It cures piles, constipation, poor eyesight, headache, deafness, colic, complexion problems and halitosis. It improves memory and students, lawyers, thinkers and all brain-workers will find it very relaxing after heavy mental work. The venous blood now flows with gravity and so the veins relax curing varicose veins. It cures loss of memory and insomnia.

Caution : Do not attempt this asana except under expert medical guidance if you happen to suffer from sinusitis, ear-ache, heart-trouble and blood pressure disorders.

CHAPTER V

BANDHAS AND MUDRAS

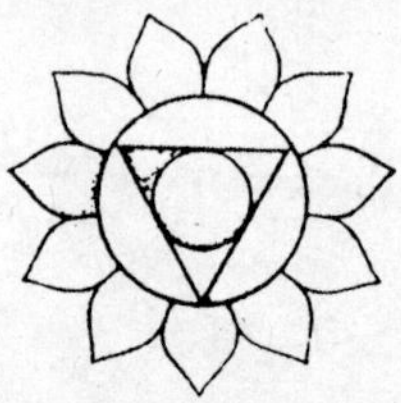

Friendship, mercy, gladness and indifference towards subjects that are happy, miserable, good and wicked respectively pacify the Chitta.

– Patanjali Yoga Sutras

Bandhas and Mudras come under the broad heading of Asanas. They are of particular value to those interested more in spiritual progress.

Most popular and widely practised is Uddayana Bandha.

1. Stand erect with the legs apart by about a foot and half.

2. Place your hands on the thighs and bring your trunk and upper half of the body forward very slightly.

3. Exhale completely.

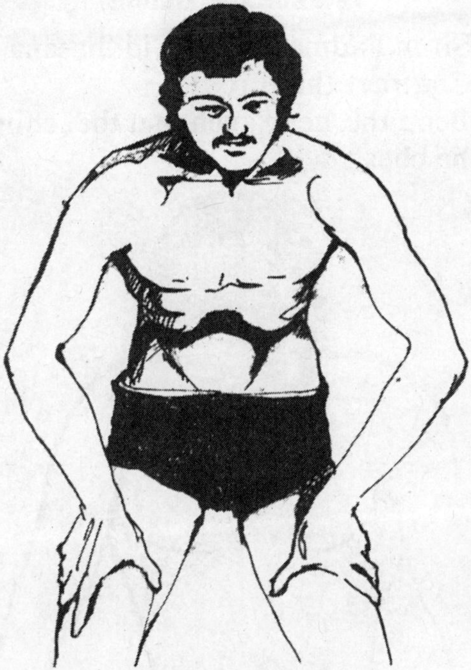

Uddayana Bandha

4. Contract your abdomen and draw up the intestines forcibly so that they are lifted up and press against the back.

5. Remain in this pose for 3-4 seconds.

6. Relax the abdominal muscles and return to the original position.

Benefits : This pose tones up the abdominal viscera and removes intestinal disorders.

Jalandhara Bandha

1. Sit in Padmasana or Siddhasana.
2. Contract the throat.
3. Bend the head such that the chin presses against the chest.

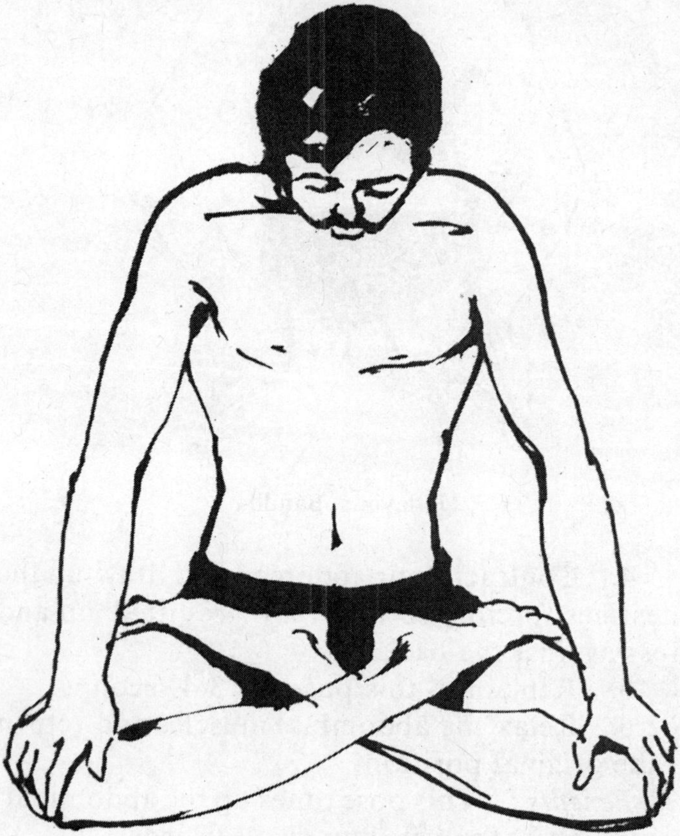

Jalandhara Bandha

4. After a few seconds, release the chin-lock.

Benefits: The thyroids are toned up and their working regulated. Giants are caused by the thyroids overworking while sluggishness of these same glands causes dwarfs. By regulating the functioning of these glands, both these unnatural conditions can be countered.

Yoga Mudra

1. Sit in Padmasana with the spine erect.

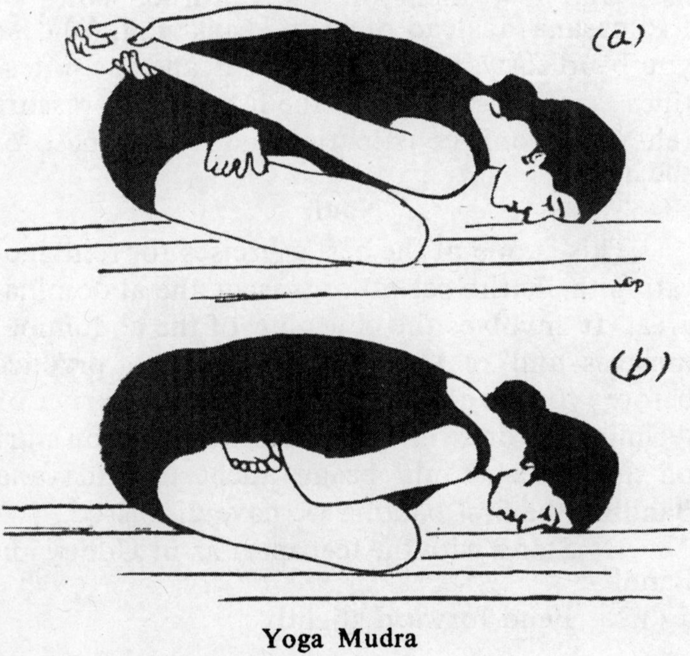

Yoga Mudra

2. Slowly bend forward until your forehead touches the ground. Exhale as you go down.

3. Take your hands behind your back and catch hold of the right wrist by the left hand Fig. (*a*).

4. Remain in this pose for 10-15 seconds.

5. Return to the original erect pose inhaling as you go up.

6. Repeat 4 times.

This mudra removes all kinds of intestinal and spleenal disorders.

A variation of this mudra is to clench the fists and rest them on the upturned soles of Padmasana instead of at the back Fig. (*b*). As you bend forward, the stomach and the intestines are pressed against the fists. This pressure relieves chronic constipation and sluggishness of the liver.

Nauli

This is one of the best exercises for reinvigorating the entire set of organs in the abdominal area. It involves the churning of the abdominal muscles and requires many months of practice before you can do it properly. This kriya or technique is done in three stages. Before you start on this, you should be an adept in Uddayana Bandha, the first bandha we have discussed.

1. Stand with the feet apart as in Uddayana Bandha.

2. Bend forward slightly.

3. Place your hands on your thighs and exhale completely.

4. Contract your abdomen and draw up your intestinal muscles so that they press against the back.

5. Now contract the abdominal muscles on both sides.

6. All the muscles will be at the centre now with hollows on either side.

This is the Central or Madhyama Nauli Fig. (*b*).

7. Relax all the muscles. Rest for a few minutes (60 seconds).

8. Do Uddayana Bandha.

9. Contract the abdominal muscles on the right side which will now look hollow. This is Right-side Nauli or Dakshina Nauli Fig. (*a*).

10. Relax all the muscles. Rest for a minute.

11. Do Uddayana Bandha.

12. Contract the abdominal muscles on the left side so that the hollow is now on this side. This is Left-side Nauli or Vama Nauli Fig. (*c*).

13. Relax the muscles and rest for a few minutes.

These kriyas cannot be done the first time but need long sustained practice. By training the abdominal muscles to contract on both sides and the centre, you will be able to contract them on whichever side you wish. Until you come to this stage, you should not venture on the next stage.

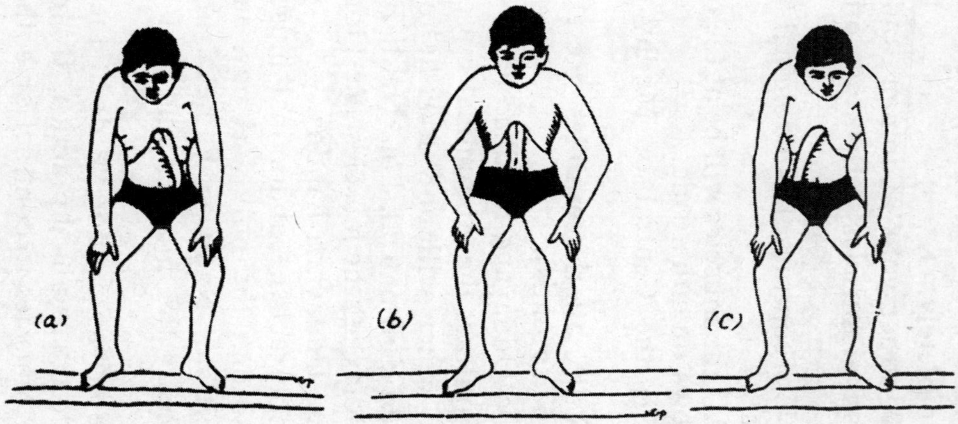

(a) Dakshina Nauli (b) Madhyama Nauli (c) Vama Nauli

After you have perfected the contraction of these muscles, first contract on the right side, next on both sides and lastly on the left side. Now again on both sides and then, the right side. These contractions must be continuous and without pausing, so that it should give the appearance of a ball rolling from side to side inside the stomach. This stage of perfection can be achieved only after practice for at least 18 to 24 months.

Benefits : This technique is the king of exercises for all disorders of the stomach, liver, spleen, pancreas, deuodenals and large intestines. The kidneys are toned up and begin to function normally.

Before you practise Uddayana Bandha and Nauli, make sure you have not eaten or drunk anything for at least 4 hours. Early morning would be the best time.

CHAPTER VI

PRANAYAMA

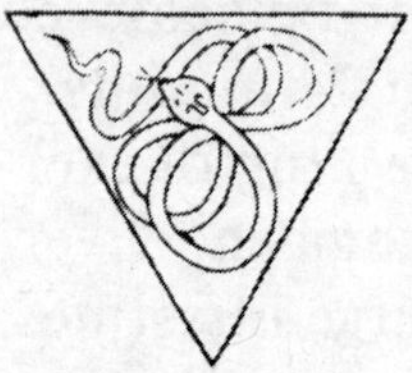

The man of well regulated endeavours controls the prana and when it has become quietened, breathes out through the nostrils. The persevering sage holds his mind as a charioteer holds the restive horses.

—Shvetashvatara Upanishad

Pranayama is the regulation or, more properly, the control of the Prana. Prana is commonly understood as breath but it is not so. It is something more vital, more subtle and powerful than breath. The English language has no equivalent for Prana. It is the universal energy or life-force that sustains the entire creation. It is found in all forms of life—animals, plants, insects, birds, organisms—and is present in every inch of space. It is the force that gives

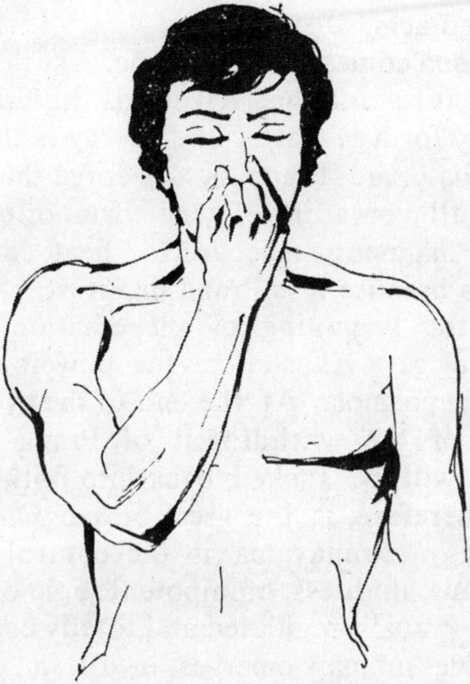

Position of Fingers during Pranayama

air its properties, man his life and water, its sustaining power. There is no single term to describe it. It is what makes the universe continue. It makes man think, feel, act, breathe and everything and anything else. Prana is the manifestation of all life and activity.

It is dormant or dynamic depending upon the stage of evolution of a man. The more evolved a person, the more dynamic and powerful is the manifestation of Prana in his thoughts, words and acts.

Akasha comes close to Prana. Akasha pervades the entire creation. All solids, liquids, gases and every form of matter and energy is the result of Akasha. And Prana is the force that makes Akasha all pervading. Every form of energy—electric, magnetic, mechanical, heat, dynamic, static—is because it is Prana manifest.

At the beginning of the creation, it was Prana that gave Akasha creative powers to bring forth the cosmos. At the end of the cycle, it is because of the withdrawal of Prana that all creation will be sucked back into nothingness. Prana, therefore, is the great power that creates everything. Pranayama is the control of this stupendous, limitless, omnipotent force or Prana. Once the Prana is regulated and totally controlled the Divine in man emerges in all its glorious powers. All men of God who have performed miracles have been able to do so because they have learnt the secret of Prana. Many realised Yogis are those who have succeeded in opening up the secrets of Prana that pervades their being. That is why a perfect Yogi becomes omnipotent. He has discovered the laws of employing Prana constructively. All people who are successful as astrologers, doctors, healers and selfless social workers are really those who have, through practice or inadvertently, stumbled upon the working of this Prana. They may or may not be aware of it. This then sums up what Prana is and that Pranayama is the control of Prana as to bring out the most constructive powers latent in a person.

There are many types of Pranayama and a book such as this cannot deal with them. Only a Guru can teach them personally.

The nervous system is closely linked with the respiratory system. You must have noticed how when a person is concentrating on a mathematical problem or when an artist is absorbed in his work, his breathing is fine and continuous without any spurts. You will also have noticed that when a man is very angry or upset or excited, he breathes heavily and shakily. This is because the state of mind is closely connected with breathing. When the mind is in a disarray, confused and worried the breathing is irregular and very little work is done. An upset man cannot do the work entrusted to him properly nor can he find a solution to the problem that is worrying him. His mind and its modifications are disorderly and moving in all directions with the sum result of zero. His breathing will also be disorderly. Conversely, if you can regulate the breathing in such a case, the mind forces will move rhythmically in one direction so that they can be constructively channelled to concentrate on the problem that requires attention. Once a person can think calmly and clearly, there is always a practical solution available, no matter what the problem is. So, we now see how closely the mind and breath are linked and with what results.

Breath becomes important because although it is not Prana, it is the most powerful manifestation of Prana in all beings. Only it has not been trained to work properly and so, man fails to cultivate the potential in him to its maximum output.

The first purpose of all Pranayama is to put order and evenness in normal breathing. This is achieved by putting aside a few minutes of everyday in your life for Pranayamic exercises.

Nadi Sodhana

This is a simple technique which gives amazing results. A minimum period of three months must be allowed before you expect results although in many cases benefits are experienced much earlier.

(1) Sit in Padmasana or Siddhasana. Keep the spine, neck and the head erect in one straight line.

(2) Close the right nostril with the thumb and inhale slowly through the left nostril

according to your capacity. Without any pause or interval, exhale slowly through the right nostril, closing the left nostril with the ring and little fingers.

(3) Again inhale through the right nostril and without any pause, exhale through the left nostril.

This completes one round of the Pranayama. The inhalation and exhalation may be unsteady and jerky in the beginning but in a week's time it will become steady and fine.

Repeat 3 rounds at one sitting with no pauses in between. The whole process must be continuous. Do it in the morning and evening. Although apparently simple, this Pranayama brings about profound changes in the mind. It gives poise and calm. It removes tension, fear and worry. It clarifies thoughts. It is a perfect and totally harmless tranquiliser. It purifies the nadis or the nervous system in about a month. In fact, even the great Adi Sankaracharya advocates this as a preliminary step to purify the nerves and before starting on other types of Pranayama. Mahayogi Aurobindo found that by the practice of Pranayama he was able to compose in half an hour, poetry that he previously could finish in a month's time. On the more worldly side, the complexion clears up and gets a dewy look. It makes the voice soft and melodious and gives lightness of the body.

Sukh Purvak

1. Sit in Padmasana or Siddhasana with head, neck and trunk erect.
2. Close the right nostril with the right thumb.
3. Inhale slowly through the left nostril, close it with the little and ring fingers.
4. Retain the breath as long as you can comfortably. At no stage, should you strain or force yourself.
5. Exhale slowly through the right nostril.
6. Again, draw in air through the right nostril, retain as in (4) and exhale through the left nostril.

This constitutes one round of the Pranayama. Repeat 3 times with a pause of 10 seconds between each round.

While inhaling think of all the beautiful qualities of love, compassion, kindness, courage, wisdom and mercy entering your being. While exhaling think that you are throwing out all the undesirable traits in your personality such as anger, hate, envy, jealousy, ill-temper, lust, avarice, etc.

After you have learnt to do this Pranayama comfortably, inhale, retain and exhale in proportional units of 1 : 4 : 2. That is, inhale for 2 counts, retain for 8 counts and exhale for 4 counts.

This Pranayama also purifies the nadis, improves clarity of thought and concentrative powers.

Bhastrika

1. Sit erect in Padmasana.
2. Inhale and exhale through both nostrils quickly and continuously about 10 times.
3. Inhale deeply and retain the breath closing both nostrils.
4. Hold the breath as long as you can comfortably without undue strain on the lungs.
5. Exhale completely.

This is one Pranayama.

6. Repeat 3 times with pauses of 15 seconds between each Pranayama.
7. Keep the mouth closed throughout. In the beginning just 4 or 5 quick inhalations and exhalations can tire you. But with practice, gradually increase the number to twenty.

This Pranayama exercises the lungs rigorously. It destroys phlegm and disorders of the respiratory canal. It supplies oxygen plentifully to the lungs. It produces heat in the body and increases appetite.

Suryabheda

1. Sit in Padmasana with the head, neck and spine held erect.

2. Close your mouth and inhale deeply through both nostrils.

3. Close your nostrils using the thumb on one side, and the little and ring fingers on the other.

4. Slowly bend your head and press your chin against your chest locking the two. (This is Jalandhara Bandha described earlier.)

5. Suck up the air in your stomach to your lungs by contracting the abdomen suddenly.

6. Retain the chin-lock and the air in your lungs for a count of 6 seconds.

7. Gradually unlock your chin from your chest exhaling slowly at the same time.

This is one Pranayama.

8. Repeat 3 times with a pause of 6 seconds between each repetition.

It stimulates the digestive system and strengthens the rib-cage and the lungs. In all Pranayama, the way you close your nostrils while retaining breath is very important. *Always use your right thumb for closing your right nostril. Use the little and ring fingers of the right hand to close the left nostril.*

Many people who do Pranayama for the first time will feel soreness of the lungs and pain in the chest-muscles. This is because all their lives, these areas will not have been exercised at all. For such people, go slowly starting with just one Pranayama per day until your chest and lungs get stronger. Very gradually, increase the number but always remember, over-enthusiasm can be disastrous. Pranayama done improperly gives pain in the ear, eyes, head, hicoughs and cough. If any of these symptoms appear, discontinue your practice and seek the aid of someone who knows all about Pranayama. According to *Hathayoga Pradeepika*, Pranayama, properly practised, can be a boon against disease but if improperly done, invites dangerous disorders of the nervous and physiological systems.

CHAPTER VII

WHAT YOU EAT

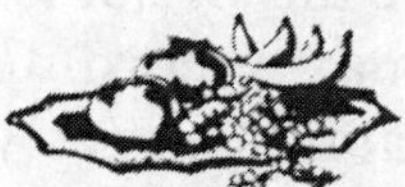

Now learn what and how great benefits a temperate diet will bring along with it. In the first place you will enjoy good health.

– **Horace**

You are what you eat. The food that goes into you influences your entire behavioral pattern. Any food you eat not only affects your physiological and organic body but also makes itself felt on your mind, nerves and thinking.

Food serves two purposes. It helps the body grow from infancy to youth to old age. It preserves the body in good health and supplies it with energy, both at the physical and mental levels.

What food does to the system can be easily understood only if we look around at Nature. The cow, a docile creature, lives on grass and husk. The tiger, which is symbolic of ferocity and rage, thrives on flesh. This does not mean a meat-free diet cannot give as much strength as a non-vegetarian diet can. The elephant, too, is a herbivore, but who can doubt its tremendous strength ? But, the elephant for all its physical strength is not wild like the tiger. It chooses to remain quiet and contented unless prodded to provocation. We can easily conclude, therefore, that food has greater influence on the mental body than on the physical body. The mind is more sensitive in its reaction to what goes into the blood and indirectly into our thoughts, which are but the product of the mind. Simple nutritious food gives a relatively clear and calm mind. Highly spiced enervating food leads to restlessness while stale food has a dulling effect on the mind.

Most cultures of the world that have survived all sorts of onslaughts have been rice-eating cultures. India, China and Japan which still today are alive and vibrant in spite of blows again and again are so only because of their thoughts. Thoughts make a man, and people make a nation. Thoughts, we have seen, are dependent on the food we eat. The highest thinkers and the most profound philosophies that have kept the people of a nation together have always originated in the East. Problems of mind and spirit with which Western nations are battling for solution, have been quietly caught by the forelock and disposed of by the Eastern philosophies.

In our own country, the ancient Rishis drew up regulations for food. These regulations were designed to bring out the Divine in the human. They were also aimed at eradicating vasanas or mental modifications which lurked in the dark recesses of the human mind, waiting for a chance to bring out the devil in him. The food invariably consisted of fruit, roots and natural products that did not involve any himsa or violence.

All food broadly comes under three categories, namely, Satwic, Rajasic and Tamasic. In order to understand this classification, we must first learn what they mean and imply. Lord Krishna deals with these three qualities in his immortal song, *The Bhagavad Gita* in Chapter 14.

Satwa, Rajas and Tamas are three qualities found in all human beings. Satwa is pure and illuminating. Rajas is differentiated by desire and craving while Tamas shows itself as delusion, ignorance, sloth and sleep.

These 3 qualities have in them the power to create certain traits in man.

When Satwa prevails, there is desire for knowledge. Cravings subside and interest is directed at leading the good life. On the other hand in a nature predominated by Rajas, the man is led on by ambition and endless desire. The main concern is sense gratification to gain which the individual constantly engages himself in action. In a Tamasic person, desire is overruled by laziness, ignorance and negative states of mind. He has no inclination to work hard but prefers to indolently waste his time and dissipate his energies.

Chapter 17 tells us how to distinguish one type of food from another.

Foods, that enhance longevity, are pure, mildly sweet or savoury, strength-giving and adding to joy, cheerfulness are Satwic. They are generally juicy and oleaginous. They tend to nourish the body and promote health. Milk and milk products, cereals, nuts, pulses, fruits, roots and vegetables are Satwic. They are not taxing on the digestive system but act to improve its working and condition.

Rajasic foods are too bitter, or sour, pungent, salty, very hot, spicy and dry and tend to promote craving in the eater. These are said to lead to disease and misery. Excessively spicy and heavy foods result in indigestion, acidity and impair the working of the digestive organs leading to ill-health. They can also create cravings which lead to involvements of every kind producing in the end misery and confusion.

Foods that are Tamasic are stale, tasteless, putrid, decayed, left-overs and unclean. Any food that is eaten later than 3 hours after it is eooked is Tamasic.

We can easily notice that most brain-workers and people who lead contented but happy lives prefer simple food that is basically Satwik. In fact, there is a saying in Tamil Nadu that from Kumbakonam hail the best brains. The expression 'Kumbakonam Iyer' is used to refer to anyone who is exceptionally intelligent and shrewd. This area comes within the rice-bowl of the South and people living here eat only rice and vegetables. Some of the best brains in the country were born in this region.

People who are in the defence and police forces, prosperous businessmen and highly successful executives caught in the rat-race of life and whose common feature is a driving ambition for victory or success are generally fond of rich, heavy foods including meat and hard drinks. This is Rajas in predominance.

Tamasic food is relished generally by the labour class which is known to eat stale food and left-overs. Unfortunately such people are neither happy nor ambitious but lead run-of-the-mill lives ruled by sloth and callousness to higher values of life.

For students of Yoga, a satwic diet is prescribed. It tends to reduce restlessness of mind at the same time providing health and strength to the body. A little meandering into dietetics becomes necessary at this stage if we are to learn the importance of food, and how different nutrients affect different functions of the body.

Dietetics

Food serves two purposes, namely, body building and maintenance of body temperature.

Proteins, minerals and water do the job of building the body and repairing damaged tissue. Carbohydrates and fat help in maintaining body temperature and producing energy for its various functions. Vitamins are necessary for the body to carry on its vital functions. Satwic food contains all these nutrients and it is not at all necessary to resort to animal food like meat, fish or eggs to keep the body strong and healthy.

Proteins make up the solid matter of muscles, organs and endocrine glands. Proteins are built of chains of amino-acids which supply the material for the building and continuous replacement of cells throughout life.

Protenis occur in rice, wheat, barley, ragi, maize, oats, nuts, milk and certain vegetables contain protein. Rice is easily digestible and cooling in effect. However, if highly polished or washed too much before cooking rice tends to constipate. Rice-eaters usually are highly intelligent. Wheat is more difficult to digest and slightly heat-producing (ushna). It helps to build the body and gives a strong and sturdy physique. It is a good substitute for rice for those suffering from diabetes. When used unpolished, it carries with it a lot of roughage which facilitates easy bowel movement. The dhals (moong, urad, bengal, horse) are very rich in protein.

Protein deficiency results in miscarriage, anaemia and premature birth. The most common affliction caused by its deficiency is kwashiorkor which occurs in infants. It also causes stunted growth and lack of resistance to infectious disease. Excess damages the kidneys.

Carbohydrates are necessary for producing energy. This energy makes use of the protein and fats to repair tissue. All starchy foods and sugar contain carbohydrates. Excess of carbohydrates can be stored in the body. It is found in rice, flour, potatoes, sweet potatoes, fruit-sugar, jaggery, all sweets and in milk. Excess of carbohydrates results in flatulence and tooth decay while its deficiency causes exhaustion, general run-down of the system and consequently ill-health.

Fats are like carbohydrates, but contain relatively less oxygen and more carbon and hydrogen. Fats are the most concentrated source of energy and in addition serve as padding around organs protecting them from shock, protect nerves, insulate the body, lubricate the intestinal tract and retard hunger. They are found in nuts, butter, milk, soyabeans, peas and in vegetable oils.

Vitamins are a necessary requirement of the body and help it to work efficiently. Vitamin deficiency results in a host of diseases and makes the system vulnerable to infection.

They were discovered late in the 19th century when a Dutch biologist Dr. Ejikman discovered that beri-beri occurred when natives ate polished rice but that could be prevented when they used rice with bran. This discovery led him to write "There is present in rice polishings a substance of a different nature from proteins, fats or salts which is essential for health and the lack of which causes nutritional polyneuritis." Vitamins cannot be cure-alls but are very necessary for certain specific body functions. Although now we have synthesised vitamins, they are best taken from Nature.

Vitamin A is fat-soluble and present in chlorophyll. It occurs in all green leaves, yellow vegetables and milk. It is found in spinach, turnips, carrots, sweet potatoes, pumpkin, apricots and cantaloupe (karbuj). This vitamin is very important for maintenance of normal vision, mucus secretions and protects against infection. It is required for skeletal and tooth development also. Deficiency causes night blindness, infections of the nasal passages and sinuses. It also causes severe drying of the skin. Supplementation of the vitamin, in the right amounts helps but excess leads to hyper-irritability, bone fragility, headaches, liver and spleen enlargement.

Vitamin B is water-soluble. It occurs in all grain-products of the whole grain variety. It is found in milk, dry beans, peas, soyabeans and peanuts. It can be lost when water in which the grain has been cooked is drained away as is the usual practice in most Indian households. Prolonged exposure to heat also leads to its loss. Its deficiency leads to beri-beri (a serious disease affecting the nerves), cramps and heaviness of the legs, paralysis of the lower limbs and emaciation. Supplementation, even in excess, is not as harmful as vitamin A because being water-soluble the excess is thrown out through urine and perspiration.

Vitamin C is also water-soluble. Synthesised vitamin C is known as ascorbic acid. It is essential for the production of material which holds the body-cells in place. It promotes the healthy development of bones, the dentine, the cartilage and connective tissues. The richest source of this is the citrus-fruit. Oranges, grape fruit, pineapples, guavas, tomatoes, lemons and sathukudi (mousambi) are very rich sources. Peaches, peas, bananas, apples, spinach, green pepper, cabbages, potatoes, sweet potatoes also contain vitamin C. This vitamin is lost by exposure to air, heat and dehydration. Especially the practice of adding baking soda while cooking is highly deplorable because although it retains the colour of the vegetable, it reduces the vitamin C level.

Deficiency of vitamin C causes scurvy characterised by tenderness and swelling of legs and thighs. It usually occurs in infants. Other symptoms of scurvy are swollen or bleeding gums, anaemia, excessive bleeding even on slight injury and bone displacement, especially in the very young. Juices of tomato and citric fruits form an excellent supplement in cases of deficiency.

Vitamin D is fat-soluble. Although it is not known how exactly this vitamin works, it is known that it regulates absorption and anchorage of calcium and phosphorus. Whenever skeletal tissue is being formed, there is need for more vitamin D. That is why expectant and nursing mothers and growing children find this vitamin so vital. Milk and sunlight are rich sources of vitamin D. Deficiency leads to infantile rickets resulting in skeletal malformations. Predisposition to dental decay and malformation of teeth are also caused by vitamin D deficiency. Milk and exposure to sunlight (only during dawn and dusk but never to the midday sun) supplement the deficiency. Ragi, a cereal common in the South, is a rich source of calcium.

Vitamin E is very necessary for carrying out the reproductive activity. It occurs in germinating wheat, rice and other seeds. Vegetables, nuts and legumes carry the vitamin in appreciable amounts.

All vitamins, proteins, carbohydrates and fats are available in Satwic form. We can use them liberally in our food to eat healthily without affecting our sadhana.

How you eat your food is no less important than what you eat. Food must be eaten with the right attitude of mind. Begin by mentally thanking God for the food you have been given (do not for a while forget how privileged you are when there are millions starving all over the world). Eat slowly. Masticate each morsel thoroughly before you swallow it. The saliva mixing with the food during the process of mastication conduces to proper assimilation of food. Otherwise, food that is not properly chewed but swallowed in haste passes through the digestive system without being assimilated and is thrown out as waste. It is better to have a glass of water by your side when you eat just in case you choke on any food. But limit intake of water to the barest minimum while eating. Too much water will dilute the digestive juices delaying and impairing proper digestion.

How much you should eat depends upon individual constitution and requirement. If you are a student or a brain-worker like a lawyer, scientist or writer you burn up food fast and need to supplement it. If you work at a job that does not require much thinking or physical movements, then you do not need as much food as in the previous cases. Growing children and expectant mothers require more food.

Generally, a student of Yoga is advised never to fill his stomach full with food. He must fill half with solid food, a quarter with water (or liquids) and leave the remaining quarter empty for air. Overfilling the stomach is over-taxing the digestive organs which may suffer a breakdown. It can also cause shortage of space for the digestive processes leading to pressure on the heart and chest pains.

The wisest thing to do is to eat moderately. As Lord Krishna says, "Yoga is not for him who eats too much or eats too little; nor for him, O, Arjuna, who sleeps too much or does not sleep enough. But for him who is moderate in food and recreation, in work and in sleep as well as in keeping awake, Yoga destroys all his sorrows."

For a Yoga student, the watchword throughout is moderation.

Food must be well-cooked and not overcooked. It must not be undercooked also. Water in which vegetables have been boiled must not be thrown away. It contains the nutritional part of the vegetable. It can be drunk as it is or used for cooking rice. Rice must not be washed too much and the water drained away because then the bran will be lost.

The gap between the two main meals can be fixed according to individual requirement but 6 hours at least would be preferable. If you have lunch at 12 in the noon, you can have supper any time after 6 in the evening. It is better you do not eat between meals but if you feel really hungry, a small snack will do no harm. But eating endlessly between meals can result in overweight problems and indigestion.

Sleeping immediately after food is not good for health. You must allow at least 3 hours after supper before you go to bed. A glass of milk after supper gives sound sleep.

Keep the dining room spotlessly clean. Hang inspiring pictures of God or saints and try to create an atmosphere of calm. Food eaten when angry, worried or upset can create ulcers and release toxins into the bloodstream.

Water

Water is life. You can live without food for as many as forty-five days but you will die in 3 days without water. Nearly 70 percent of the body weight is of water. Perspiration and urination deplete the body of liquid which must be constantly replenished.

The body requires at least 8 glasses of water daily to make up for losses in various ways. Drinking during eating has to be minimised. Water can be drunk at least 2 hours after or before a meal. Otherwise it intereferes with the digestion. A glass of water first thing on rising and just before going to bed sets right elimination problems. In fact, keeping the water in a copper pot or mug for some hours before drinking is recommended in cases of severe constipation.

Water at room temparature is best. But sometimes when it has to be boiled due to either a person being ill or municipal instructions, cool it thoroughly and pour it slowly from one vessel to another several times. This process replaces the prana eliminated while boiling the water.

Water is used in Nature Cure. This is called Hydrotherapy and is very effective. Water packs are used for fighting fevers. Three or four blankets are spread on the floor. Over them is spread a wet bedsheet which has been wrung dry. The patient lies on this sheet. The sheet and blankets are wrapped round him. Very soon, he begins to sweat and the temperature comes down to normal.

The hip-bath also helps in fever. The patient sits in a tub of water. The parts of his body outside the tub are kept covered and warm. The abdomen is massaged with a coarse or rough towel for about 20 minutes when the temperature begins to fall. Water baths, in themselves, are invigorating and refreshing. A daily bath is very important for personal hygiene. Reasonably warm water is suited for the average man. The bath must be followed by vigorous rubbing with a dry towel so that circulation improves.

Splashing the eyes with cold water every morning keeps them cool and healthy.

Fasting

Fasting was prescribed as a universal remedy in ancient times. 'Langhanam Paramoushadham' said the ayurvedic doctors. A fast every week or fortnight gives the digestive system a much needed rest. At the same time it gives the body a chance to cleanse itself of accumulated toxins. Plenty of water must be taken during a fast. It flushes the system of obstinate waste-matter and prevents excessive acidity in the stomach.

You can set aside a particular day at regular intervals of times for a fast. It can be a total fast when you eat or drink nothing except plain water. Or, you can take only liquids such as buttermilk, milk and fruit juice. Stimulants like tea and coffee are best avoided, because they tend to stimulate the central nervous system when your intention is to give yourself a rest. Fasts, longer than a day, require supervision under a competent guide and it is better you do not venture on them by yourself.

Wc have learnt so much about food but if you ask me 'What is the right diet ?' I cannot still give you any answer. There can be no one right diet. The best answer would be to first find out everything about health conditions and your problems and then draw up a suitable diet-programme. If you still insist, I can only suggest more vegetables, more fruits and milk and less starchy and fried foods. And plenty of fresh cool (but not chilled or iced) water in between meals. Less coffee and tea. Most diseases can be safely handled and brought under control by altering your dietary habits.

It was not for nothing that Hippocrates said, "*Thy food shall be thy remedy*".

A young lady of about 27 years once came to me about her eyes. I noticed she was impeccably dressed and wore mod glasses, large curved lenses set in gold rims. She could not see well in dim light. She was a working girl and so could only go to the night shows of which she was quite fond. She dreaded going to the theatre with her friends for fear they would discover her defect. She would invariably fall behind them trying to find her way in the dark. She could see the rows only with difficulty and never failed to step on people's toes or sit right on top of them not being able to make out if the seat was empty or not in the darkness of the auditorium. She was quite unhappy over her night-blindness. The first thing I asked her to do was to get rid of her mod glasses and wear instead smaller lenses. The mod glasses were unduly curved causing strain on the eyes. I then told her she must cut down on all fried, pasty, starchy foods which she really loved and include instead in her daily diet raw carrots and some greens, raw or cooked. I also advised her to give up reading while lying down. When she came back to see me again a year later, she reported not only better vision but a better complexion as well. There were no costly visits to the opticians or no high sounding drugs. Just supplementation of vitamin A and correction of a faulty habit and diet.

A happy blending of Yogasanas, Pranayama, attitudes (Yama and Niyama) and regulated diet can make your life happier, healthier and more meaningful.

CHAPTER VIII

WHAT YOGA CAN DO

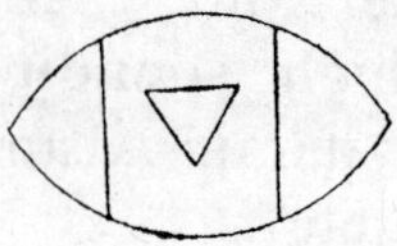

Yoga succeeds by the six (qualifications)—zeal, bold determination, courage, true knowledge, firmness and renunciation of the company of unsuitable people.

—**Hathayogapradipika.**

Innumerable women from all walks of life and of all ages have found remarkable benefits by following yogic techniques I have taught them. Young girls, teenagers, middle-aged women and even those who have retired from active life have come to me with woes of all sorts and after completing my course of Yoga have come out of the Institute smiling, relieved and feeling totally rejuvenated. My own experience in dealing with hundreds of ladies has taught me to judge each case as unique. This rules out, therefore, any general technique of yogasanas and pranayama. I modify the technique (asana, pranayama, or dhyana) to answer the specific needs of each case which entails individual attention. Several frustrated ladies who have tried all types of medication—allopathy, ayurvedic, nature cure and even surgery in some instances and have been disgusted with their 'incurable problems' of health and mind have come to me as a last resort. Just 3 months of carefully planned and programmed courses in yoga have given them such astonishing results, that they have been quite overwhelmed by this simple yet sure remedy. Grateful letters from them testify to the amazing benefits of proper yogic therapy.

(1) Piles and Asthma

Dear Mathaji,

I am very happy to write about my unforgettable experience in my life at this institute. I had been suffering from piles and allergic asthma for several years. There was no treatment that I did not try to cure these diseases. But all in vain. I was very worried and there was no mental rest for me. Luckily, I was introduced to this institute where I was trained in meditation and Yoga exercises. These have given me much mental peace and a disciplined life to lead. The diet that has been suggested to me has given me relief from my complaints.

I pay my humble respects and I shall ever remain grateful. to this institute and Mathaji.

Yours sincerely,
Indira Krishnaswamy.

(2) Diabetes

A middle-aged housewife, the wife of an eminent political figure in Karnataka, underwent the course and found herself completely cured of diabetes. She writes :

Dear Smt. Guruji.

First of all, I thank you very much for your kind guidance in the practice of Yoga. This has helped me a lot. I am now completely cured of diabetes.

Yours faithfully,
Y. P. Channabasamma.

(3) Blood Pressure, Piles, Varicose Veins

For twenty years, the wife of a businessman suffering from painful piles, varicose veins and low blood pressure found relief by practising Yoga. She writes :

Dear Guruji Rajeswari,

I am very glad to inform you that after joining the Yoga classes and practising it regularly according to your instructions, I have completely recoverd from piles trouble, from which I was suffering for the last twenty years. There is no sign of piles at all now. The blood pressure, which always used to be low, is now normal. Before I was very short tempered and this has also decreased to some extent. Before joining the Yoga classes, I had started to bulge out day-by-day, which also subsided. On the contrary, I have even lost some weight. I was suffering from varicose veins—even that has decreased. I am most thankful to Guruji, as it is not only Yoga that helps us, but more than that, we require the blessings of the Guru. No one has seen God, but I see God in my Guruji. God never helps us directly, but through some mediator and I am sure Guruji is a mediator.

Yours sincerely,
Veena Shrichand.

More people than we can imagine seem to suffer from piles. Usually, this is because of faulty elimination, although there can be other reasons too. Yoga, properly practised, tones up the eliminatory system which is the first requisite for good health.

(4) Eczema

Skin afflictions are caused by glandular irregularities. Certain yogic techniques perform the job of setting them right. Eczema, characterised, by scaly formations on the skin, wet or dry, can be both embarrassing and uncomfortable if it starts to itch.

My dear Guru Mrs. Rajeswari Raman,

I have been a great sufferer from eczema. The disease was more severe when I went abroad. Under your training I am practising certain yogic exercises. I had great difficulty in doing this at first, but after some days' effort I succeeded. Now, I am most happy to state that I have recovered almost totally from this disease. Apart from this, my general health has also improved to a large extent.

Yours sincerely,
Bharati.

(5) Anger, Breathlessness and Overweight

Dear Guruji,

I would like to give the following report after having undergone the Yoga course in your institute.

When my friend Chandrika joined the course, she also wished that I should join. But some people scared me saying that it was dangerous. I do not till now know what they meant by it.

About six months back, I started to put on weight. In addition to this, I also found I was getting angry and had become very short tempered and for trifle things I used to shout and flare up.

To reduce my weight, I started consulting doctors who prescribed various medicines and gave diet charts which were of no use at all. At this time, my friend Chandrika advised me to join your Yoga school to get a proportionate figure.

After learning Yoga under you, I really do feel that it was wise of me to have joined the course. I feel it has made me realise that Yoga is the training of the physical body and the mental faculties to become steady, alert and potent to change their nature and to remove obstacles in the way and realise the true nature of the Self.

I have been able to control my temper and do not get angry nowadays. I do hope as time passes on, I will be able to win over my anger completely and also get a good proportionate figure. If I climbed stair-cases or walked fast, my breathing used to become quicker, but now after learning Yoga, I never feel tired to walk long distances even. I am really glad I joined Sri Suryaprakash Institute of Yoga.

Yours truly,

L. M. Prabhavati.

(6) Obesity and Mental Calm

Dear Respected Guruji,

I have learnt that the human body and mind need exercise to be in a good condition and 'Yoga' is the best form of exercise. By learning Yoga the scientific way, I have been able to keep my body flexible and my mind clear.

Before I started on the Yoga course, I was short-tempered, I had extra weight and was having a considerable waist line. But now I have cut down my weight by 3 Kgs. and my waist line by 8 cms. and I have also control over my temper. I get sound s eep and have peace of mind.

I agree with the fact that 'Yoga' is a must for everyone young or old to build up and keep a beautiful, proportionate, strong and healthy body with sound mental health.

Yours faithfully,

Mrs. K. S. Vijayalakshmi.

(7) Sinus Trouble, Social Adjustment and Tension

Respected Guruji,

I find Yoga simple in technique, easy to practise and non-tiring. It gives me a lot of energy. I do not feel tired even after working for eight hours in school.

My headache and sinus trouble have completely disappeared.

I have achieved more self-confidence, better behaviour and social adjustment.

Yoga has helped me a lot in reducing stress, tension and worry. And a sense of well-being pervades me.

M. S. Chanpaka Malini.

(8) Flexion of Knee and Mental Upliftment

My beloved Guruji,

Here is a brief report of my condition both prior to as well as after a course in Yoga.

I met with an accident on 4–1–1974 with an extensive wound on and around my right knee, a fracture of the thigh bone at the middle of the right leg. The wound was sutured under general anaesthesia and a blood transfusion given.

As this sutured wound did not heal and there was falling of the wound cover, *i.e.*, the skin (they treated it as open wound for 2 months and 20 days later), they removed the skin from the left leg and grafted it to the wound on the right leg under general anaesthesia. My bone had healed up wrongly shortening my right leg by 3 inches.

So, they broke the union and inserted a steel rod inside the bone to keep both the cut ends in opposition. This was the major operation. After 15 days I was sent home.

This total period lasted 5 months and 20 days during which I had to lie down on my back. I could not bend my leg. I used to sit stretching my leg. While climbing steps I had to use one leg at a time dragging the other to the same step like a child does.

Added to it, the steel rod inserted was long and protruding which could be felt under the skin. It was giving me a lot of pain in movement of limb and joint. I started on clutches. Because of non-usage, the muscles on my leg, especially below my knee, shrank up.

In spite of repeated requests for advice at the Government Hospital for further guidance they turned me out.

Unable to bear the pain I approached a reputed physiotherapist of Bangalore. Within 20 days of attendance, I was driven to a conclusion that I must end my life, because of the pain I had to tolerate by the manual force used in his treatment for bending. Added to that there was that protruding nail under my skin. I began to get pains in my ears, head and neck because of the pain caused by the forceful bending. It continued to be as painful on the day after the intramodullary bone pinning, that is insertion of the steel rod.

I decided to go to St. Martha's Hospital in order to get this nail out. But they drove the nail deeper because there was no firm union of the cut and end of the bone.

I was advised physiotherapy at St. Martha's. Even after 10 days there was no improvement of flexion of knee beyond 30°. So I continued to limp. To my ill-luck they advised me to undergo another operation on my knee promising only 90° flexion, (bending of knee) but which would also mean that my knee would remain weak henceforth. I got alarmed because as it was I had the replaced tissue on my knee instead of the original skin. This replaced tissue does not work like the original.

Cursing God for having saved me on the day of the accident, I decided to get discharged from the hospital and flee from doctors.

I started screening for professional masseurs at the Government Ayurvedic Hospital and other places. The so-called masseurs were reluctant to touch my leg because of extensive replaced tissue around the knee. I searched even at Nelamangala and other places and went on paying money for the oils they supplied.

Meanwhile I met one masseur who was much better than the physiotherapist in the sense that my leg started bending at the knee from 30° to to 65°. But there was much pain to endure.

And I still had to sit stretching my right leg and limp. I could not carry any weight on this limb. Meanwhile my bone had set properly and I wanted to get my bone pin, *i.e.*, the steel rod, out, as it was preventing the movement of my right hip joint. I got admitted to St. Martha's Hospital again. The calcium deposit around the steel rod was so much they had to bore 5 holes in it to loosen and remove it.

The whole process of walking on crutches followed by a walking stick had to be done with the dreaded fear of a weak bone inside. I got exhausted both physically and mentally because of this endurance test for 14 long months.

The doctors advised me to continue at the masseur. I had flexion of my leg only to 65°. I still continued to limp. I was unable to sleep on my right side. I lived with pain.

I am a veternary doctor working with large animals. This profession gave me much satisfaction, but after the accident I was deprived of this.

After taking a course in Yoga under you, I have achieved much through your gentle care which I shall list out.

(1) I can sit cross-legged.

(2) I can walk normally.

(3) My bending of knee has reached 120°.

(4) I did not get any pain during Yoga practice. Moreover, I started feeling light.

(5) Gay, active: This mental transformation was within a span of $1\frac{1}{2}$ months.

(6) My pain in the ear, back of head and neck has vanished.

(7) I can organise my thinking.

(8) I am no longer irritable.

(9) I do not feel lonely.

(10) I use one leg for each step either to climb or to come down like any normal person.

(11) I can sit cross-legged throughout the time of dhyana and pranayama.

(12) You have rehabilitated me to my almost normal self except for a little more of flexion of the knee.

(13) Added to everything I have escaped that dreaded operation on my knee for flexion. I have now a strong knee which is yielding day after day.

I am sure that I will soon be back at my work at the Hospital and return to that satisfactory life. It is a new life and outlook to life you have given me.

Ma, all the worldly knowledge is so insignificant in front of this great "Yoga", which can relieve pain and human suffering. Each human being who looks to you for help will go happy and remain great throughout his life.

I, as your student, will remain grateful to you and pray God to give you all happiness and prosperity on earth.

I wish many more who are handicapped like me will come to you for your gentle care. You are a source of help, peace and greatness.

Your ever loving child,
Dr. N. Vinuthamani.

(9) Migraine and Menstrual Disorder

Respected Smt. Rajeswari Raman Guruji,

After having attended the Yoga class for four weeks, I feel that my periods are now becoming regular, *i.e.*, I am having my periods within two months. I feel light and gay. I used to get migraine headache once in 7 days. Now I get it once in 15 days. I was weighing 157 lbs. when I joined the course. Now I weigh 152 lbs. My skin colour is slowly changing. I have more peace of mind. I feel much more confident and happy.

Yours faithfully,
Nagaratna Niranjan.

(10) Irregular Menstruation

Guruji,

I am doing Yoga as per your instructions. After doing Yoga I feel light and fresh and active throughout the day. I have lost a pound in weight. As a result I have gained some self-confidence in which I was lacking earlier. I had pain in my back and hips which are disappearing gradually. Irregular menses are becoming regular after learning Yoga.

Your obedient student,
Padmavathi, R.

(11) Nervous Tension and Depression

My dearest Guruji,

It is a pleasure to write about my experience in Yoga classes. I came here with problems like depression, lack of self-confidence, disinterest in work and consequently a feeling of putting off all my work which would get me so worked up that the situation was leading me to a nervous breakdown. Since I do not like resorting to drugs, these problems together with pain in the limbs were bothering me for a long time. Fortunately I got the opportunity of joining this Institute and I came here almost as a patient going to a doctor. Now after about three months of regular training and personal attention given by you this 'Nature Cure' is gradually working on me and I feel I am seventy percent better. I am sure I will be a perfectly normal person with regular practice in future, and your blessings. Hence, my dear Madam, you have got the honour of making me more useful to the field in which I am working.

To elaborate my experience--most scientifie people may not believe in meditation which is taught here first. But I, as an Engineer, can say that this has got scientific value since it teaches us to concentrate our mind which medicine cannot. When we close our eyes and repeat 'OM', this Omkara has got such a wonderful effect on our nervous system that we feel as if we have got extra strength. When we open our eyes after 'Pranayama', we feel our eyes to be very fresh. And also about each pose of Yoga that has been taught here I feel as if I have achieved something. In this modern world of maddening rush and unhealthy competition everywhere, it is this Yoga which gives peace of mind which is very essential for health. And also I have no fear now of becoming fat and I can eat what I like.

Before closing this letter, kindly permit me to write a few lines about you—my dear Guruji. I found a great lady in you dedicating yourself for the good of others without expecting any reward. The way you treat your students has a healing effect. You have poured motherly affection on me and you will remain in my memory for ever. The only way I think of rewarding you is to offer my sincerest prayers to God to give you a long, healthy, happy life.

I am rather sorry to leave this place, but I have to and I do so, requesting my Guruji—Mrs. Rajeswari Raman—to kindly remember me as one of her disciples.

Dr. (Miss) T. S. Vedavathy,
Indian Institute of Science.

(12) Reinvigoration

Dear Guruji,

I am really grateful to you for all that you have taught me. Yoga of course is a wonderful thing, but I have gained something more. Your meditation has really put me on the right path. How I enjoy my meditation now as this is connected with Yoga! I am so fond of Yoga, I cannot proceed until I do the meditation. So I have learnt two things, one meditation, and the other, Yoga. So, you can imagine, how happy I feel. You are really doing wonderful work for humanity. May God give you long life to live and help people benefit more and more from you.

I may add that I have been a keen sportswoman; riding, swimming and tennis have been my regular games, but I can tell you before your Yoga, these things are nothing.

Wishing you all the best,

Yours sincerely.
Shanta Choudhri,
w/o of the Retd. I.G. of Police,
Delhi.

(13) Mental and Emotional Tensions

Dear Guruji,

I am most grateful to you for teaching me Yoga which has helped me tremendously.

I feel physically fit and mentally happy now. My worries and mental tensions have decreased to a great extent. I also feel very active throughout the day—that feeling of laziness has gone completely. I can control my temper and emotions whenever I want to now. In short I feel quite light in body and mind. My occasional backaches have disappeared too.

A million thanks to you Guruji.

Yours obediently,
Rama Bali.

(14) Falling Hair, Rashes and Mental Exhaustion

Dear Respected Guruji,

The effect of Yoga on my mental and physical conditions is really inexpressible. Before joining the Yoga Institute, I had a sort of nervous tension in the left side of my head, neck and limbs. I was getting measle-like rashes all over the body. My mental condition was so horrible, my mind refused to do any work. I was not getting sleep and my hair was falling. After learning Yoga, all my troubles have started lessening day by day. After doing Pranayama the rashes have disappeared almost completely, my memory power has increased and my intelligence seems to be getting sharpened which is very important for a research worker like me. After doing other Yogic poses my nervous tension has decreased considerably and I get sleep. I hope all my troubles will be cured completely if I continue to do Yoga every day. The treatment that I received from you was so wonderful I simply fail to express it in words. I have immense pleasure in writing that this treatment has given me extra strength and interest in learning Yoga. The meditation that you taught me has not only influenced the moral aspect but also the spiritual aspect of my life.

You are the first "Great Lady" in my life and have impressed me so much. You are dedicating your life solely for the benefit of others without expecting any reward. For the motherly treatment, the sincere training and everything that you have poured on me, I am grateful to you all my life. I only wish that my unfortunate sisters who are suffering like me will come in contact with you and get relieved of their trouble.

The pleasure of my association with you is just unforgettable and I will be eagerly looking forward for a call from you in case I am needed for some service at your place.

Yours faithfully,
T. S. Rukmini,
Research Student,
Indian Institute of Science,
Bangalore–12.

(15) Muscular Pains in the Chest

Dear Mrs. Raman,

When I had the very great pleasure of an interview with your husband last May, he advised me that special Pranayama would be of help to me in connection with chest pains from which I have suffered for a number of years past, and which he predicted might well become worse as the years go by. Several doctors whom I have consulted about these pains have told me that they are muscular and that I would have to put up with them since they were inside my chest.

After my interview with your husband, I had the pleasure of meeting you when you taught me Pranayama different from that which I have been practising for the last 20 years or so, also a different form of meditation. I have practised both ever since the day I met you, and am happy to say that my chest pain has left me. In addition, I feel much better both mentally as well as physically as a consequence. I spend between 15 to 20 minutes every morning on Pranayama and 25 to 30 minutes on meditation.

I am writing this letter because I would like you to know how grateful I am to you for giving me such beneficial help.

With kind regards,

Yours sincerely,
Cecil Stack,
Hertfordshire (U.K.).

(16) Colitis

I congratulate Mrs. & Mr. B. V. Raman for initiating me in Pranayama for a cure of my colitis. Sometime ago when I was much upset with persistent stomach disorder and in spite of all medical assistance I could not get relief, I happened to meet Mr. Raman at my garage. When I told him of my ailments, he asked me to meet him at his residence. When I met him accordingly he advised me to take to 'Pranayama' regularly and instructed Mrs. Raman to teach me the same and to put me in the way. Under the able guidance of Mrs. Raman, I am glad to say, I started to do 'Pranayama' and continued the course of exercise for over three months. Now I am quite free from my stomach disorders. I take this opportunity to thank Mrs. and Mr. Raman once again, for their able guidance.

P. Damodaram.

(17) Bleeding Piles and Constipation

Respected Guruji,

I had little knowledge of Yoga before coming to you. I suffered very much due to constipation which developed into bleeding piles. I had to undergo surgery twice in my life and thought I might be subjected to further operations. This disturbed me to a great extent mentally and physically. It was really my good fortune to come to you. I am completely relieved of my trouble now. The Yoga techniques with spiritual outlook, especially meditation and concentration, have benefited me considerably. The lecture given by you on the opening day of the session was a very appealing one. I believe that I will achieve that will-power in my future life and follow Yama, Niyama etc. I shall try and endeavour to stop mind-wandering and I am sure I will succeed gradually in my effort. As a wife and mother and having closer attachment to the family than my husband I required greater efficiency and resoluteness of the mind in my daily life and the Yoga taught by you has offered me an ideal training for physical and mental efficiency.

My daughter, Anuradha who is also your student, suffered much from respiratory troubles. Now she is relieved of her troubles under your care.

I remain ever grateful to you for all the benefits your Yoga classes have bestowed on me and I pray that your Institution may continue to grow and develop for imparting training to more and more women who are ailing both mentally and physically. I and my daughter thank you very much for the kindness and effective guidance given to us.

Yours affectionately,
M. V. Godavari.

(18) Improvement in Voice and Chronic Backache

Dear Gurudev,

I write this letter with great pleasure after the completion of the Yoga course under your kind guidance. I would also like to place on record that the course has immensely helped to improve my health in general and the following in particular.

(*a*) My chronic backache has been nearly cured.

(*b*) There has been a distinct improvement in my voice during singing.

With highest of regards,

Yours sincerely,
Smt. Kanta Chandra.

(19) Over-Pigmentation of Skin and Temper

Dear Guruji,

.........I was suffering from over-pigmentation for over 3 years or so. Even though I took medicine I could not find any improvement but so soon after I started the Yoga course under you, I find my skin becoming fairer and smoother than before.

........I have become more beautiful and I find my body is very light. I feel I have become strong. I have started doing my work without grumbling. I do not lose my temper now like before........

Your faithful student,
Shila, M. S.

(20) Burning in Legs and Sleeplessness

Respected Guruji,

I was suffering from shooting pain and burning sensation of my right leg–thigh, knee and upto the foot completely for the last two years. There was swelling too. I could not bend it in the normal manner. The shooting pains used to occur intermittently and irregularly. As a result, I had to spend sleepless nights. I had lost appetite....I was getting peevish. My monthly courses were irregular. My entire health was upset and broke down. Almost everyday in the evening I used to get fever.

I consulted a number of doctors and used many medicines prescribed by them. But all were of no avail. At last even the bone specialist came to the inevitable conclusion that as a last resort my leg had to be operated upon.

At that stage 'Yoga Abhyasa' in your institution under your kind directions was suggested by one friend....for the last 3 months I have been regularly practising the Asanas kindly taught by you, as per your directions strictly. Now I am very glad to say that within this short period I have found remarkable improvement in my health. All my ailments have become almost extinct. The shooting pain and burning sensation have almost disappeared. I get sound sleep. I feel good normal appetite. The physical appearance has improved a lot. Periodicity in menses has set in. I am now sober....Now I have completely stopped taking any medicine and have taken to regular practice (of Yoga) as directed by you.

Yours faithfully,
Padma Narayanaswamy.

(21) Long-standing Pain in Leg and Weight Reduction

Dear Guruji,

After I started doing Yoga I have recovered completely from the long-standing pain I was suffering in my left leg. Pre-menstrual and menstrual pains have also disappeared. I have lost 3 pounds. There is overall improvement in physical and mental health.

Sincerely yours,
Nalini B. Bhat.

(22) Numbness in Hands and Gas Trouble

Dear Guruji,

....First I had numbness in my hands. Now I am completely cured of that. I had gas trouble also and that also, I feel, has gone....With Pranayama I feel very fresh and happy. I get peace of mind.

Yours faithfully,
Visalakshi Natarajan.

(23) Sinusitis, Menstrual Regulation and Improved Vision

Dear Madam,

I have been almost cured of sinusitis—an ailment which used to trouble me at fairly frequent intervals. My menstrual cycle of 40 days has been partially corrected to 35 days. My vision has improved and I am generally more alert and active. The diet suggested by Mrs. Raman together with the asanas has helped me reduce my weight. I indeed have much to thank Mrs. Raman for my improved physical health and less irritable temperament.

Sukanya Rathnam.

(24) Bronchitis, Hip and Body Pain

Respected Madam,

I had bronchitis trouble for the past 3 years. I thought that my disease would not be cured at all and I would have to take medicines for the rest of my life. During winter how I would suffer....and long for sleep....Now I get sound sleep. I get the attack now and then but not at all severe....I no longer get body and hip pain which I used to get before....You take so much pains to make others happy.

Yours faithfully,
Thilakavathi C.G.

(25) Stomach Cramps, Giddiness and Irritability

My Dear Respected Guruji,

I was frequently getting severe cramps, giddiness and I was easily irritable. You were kind enough to listen to my woes, took me as your student, imparted to me the knowledge of Yoga and relieved me of my maladies....

Yours obediently,
Narmada Simha.

(26) Deuodenal Ulcers

Respected Guruji,

I was a patient of deuodenal ulcers and I used to take 'Gelucil' pills daily. Soon after taking to Yoga, I have discontinued the drug. Now I feel that I am free of that trouble. Mentally also I used to be very short-tempered. I am improved mentally also.

Yours obediently,
N. Kanthamani.

(27) Arthritis

Dear Guruji,

I was suffering from severe pain in the knee-joint due to arthritis. I was not able to sit down on the floor for long. In spite of doing Yoga rather irregularly, I have derived two benefits : I am now able to sit without much discomfort on the floor and pain in joints is much less these days. I am full of hope of a complete cure if I strictly follow your instructions both in the techniques of Yoga and diet.

Your grateful student,
Dr. Ratna N. Shriyan.

(28) Migraine and Lung Congestion

Dear Guruji,

The terrible migraine headache that I was suffering from has disappeared completely. My lungs which were congested seem to be clearer. I have reduced in weight by 8 pounds. I weighed 114 lbs. before. Now I weigh only 106 lbs.

Yours sincerely,
Prema Krishnan.

(29) Gain in Height and Weight

Dear Guruji,

I started doing Yoga on 16th May 1974 and the results as on 6th July 1974 are too good to believe. Previously I weighed 34.5 Kgs. Now I weigh 38 Kgs. I have gained 5 cms. height as well in the past one month....In the past 10 years I have tried all the tonics and drugs available in the City but none of them ever helped me. Within a period of 50 days you have helped as no doctor ever has or ever will....

Yours very sincerely,
Mallika Subramanyam.

(30) Asthma and Allergy

Respected Guruji,

I have pleasure in expressing hearty thanks to you for giving me training in certain Yogic exercises which have given miraculous results to my allergic asthma from which I was suffering since 6 months. Prior to joining the Yoga class, even a little milk-curds and some kinds of vegetables and fruits used to cause asthma. Within 2 months of Yoga exercises, I feel much healthier and I can enjoy all the eatables which I was allergic to earlier.

Yours most sincerely,

Lachmi Devidas.

SRI SURYA PRAKASH INSTITUTE OF YOGA FOR WOMEN

Verily, O Son o Pritha, there is destruction for him, neither here nor hereafter, for the doer of good never comes to grief.

– Srimad Bhagavad Gita.

The Object

At the suggestion of well-meaning friends, this Institute was started for imparting to women simple Yoga techniques which could be of immense benefit to their physical and mental well-being.

What Yoga Means ?

There is a feeling that Yoga is something mysterious and out of reach to the average person. This is not a correct view. Yoga in common parlance may be defined as a process of ensuring a perfect balance between bodily functions and thought-processes taking into account that a human being lives at various phases of life—physical, mental, emotional and spiritual—simultaneously.

What Yoga Can Do ?

Yoga enables one to be free from physical breakdown, mental fatigue and emotional imbalance, apart from its spiritual objective. It equips the man or woman with the technique of catching happiness and it can make one's life pleasant and enjoyable.

Who Can Learn Yoga ?

Irrespective of caste, creed, race, religion, nationality or sex, everyone can learn Yoga under a proper teacher.

Yoga is a boon to women of all ages—young, old, middle-aged, mothers, housewives, working women, artistes, musicians, etc., to secure and preserve a healthy and active body and to overcome physical ailments and mental and emotional disturbances.

Young women can acquire and keep up attractive figures and avoid corpulence.

Those suffering from stomach-upsets, uterine troubles, migraine, back-ache, tension, nervousness, exhaustion, weariness of body, body pains, etc., can derive immense benefit.

Course in Yoga

Based on ancient texts and her own experience, Mrs. Rajeswari Raman has devised a course of Yogic Sadhana—Asanas, Pranayama, meditation, etc., for the benefit of women.

The duration of the course is about three months. Those interested may contact Mrs. Rajeswari Raman on the telephone any day between 12 noon and 1 p.m. (Phone : 34078) for an appointment or write to Mrs. Rajeswari Raman, "Sri Rajeswari", 115/1, New Extension, Seshadripuram, Bangalore 560 020.

PLATES

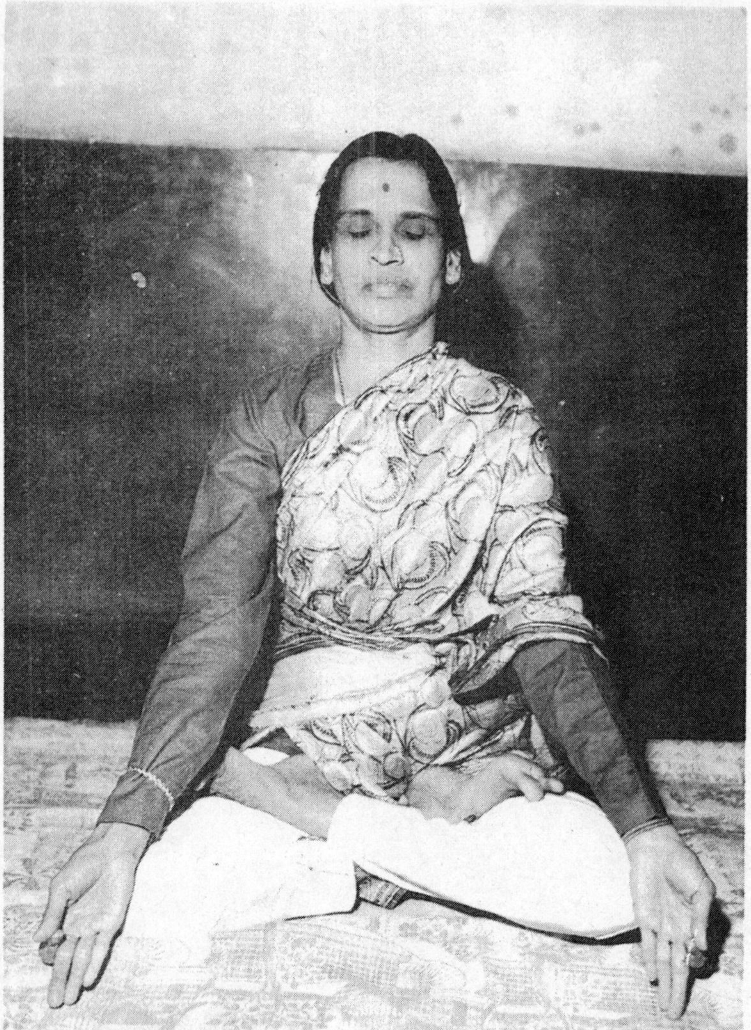

Padmasana

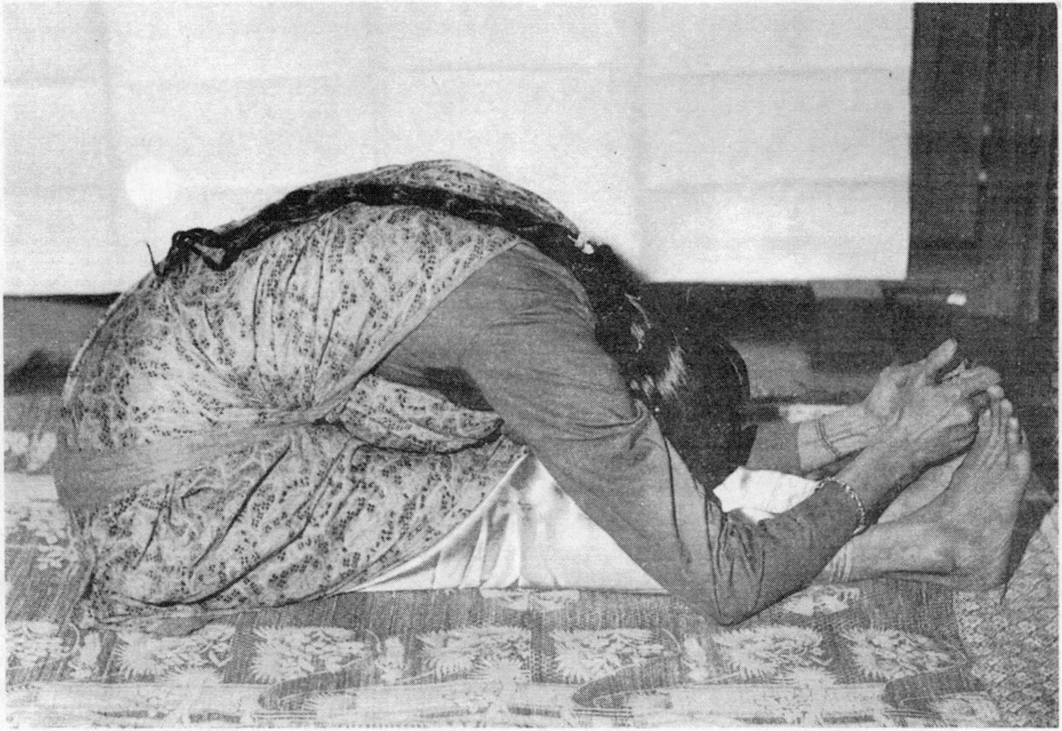

Paschimuttanasana

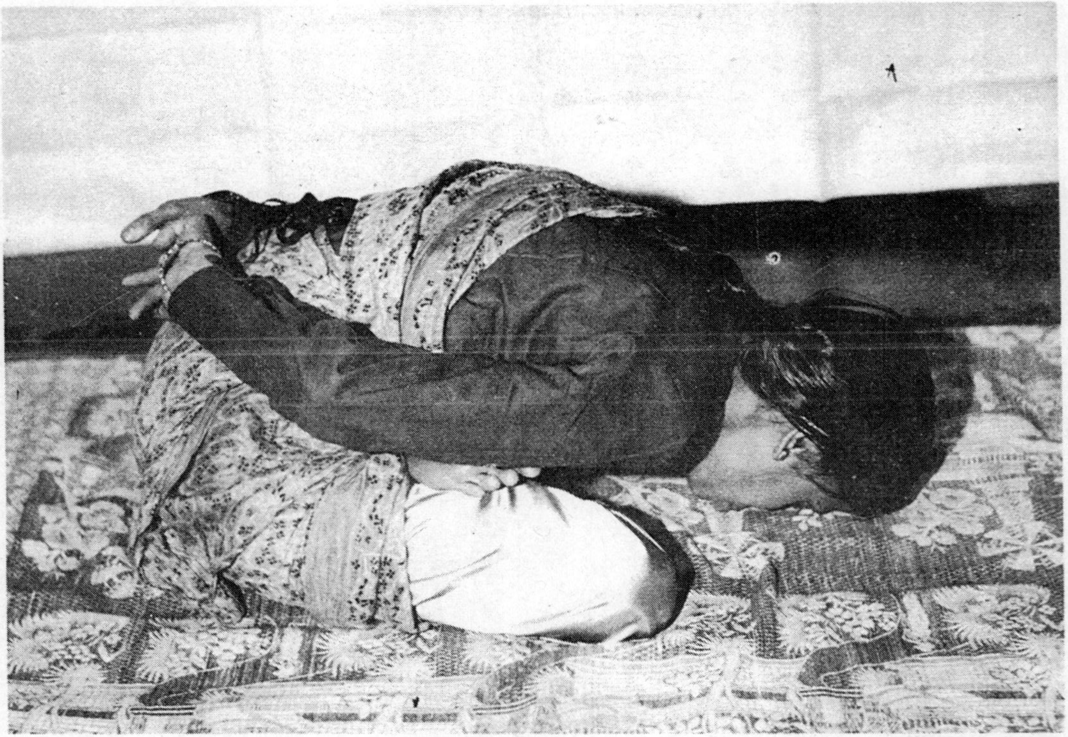

Yoga-mudra

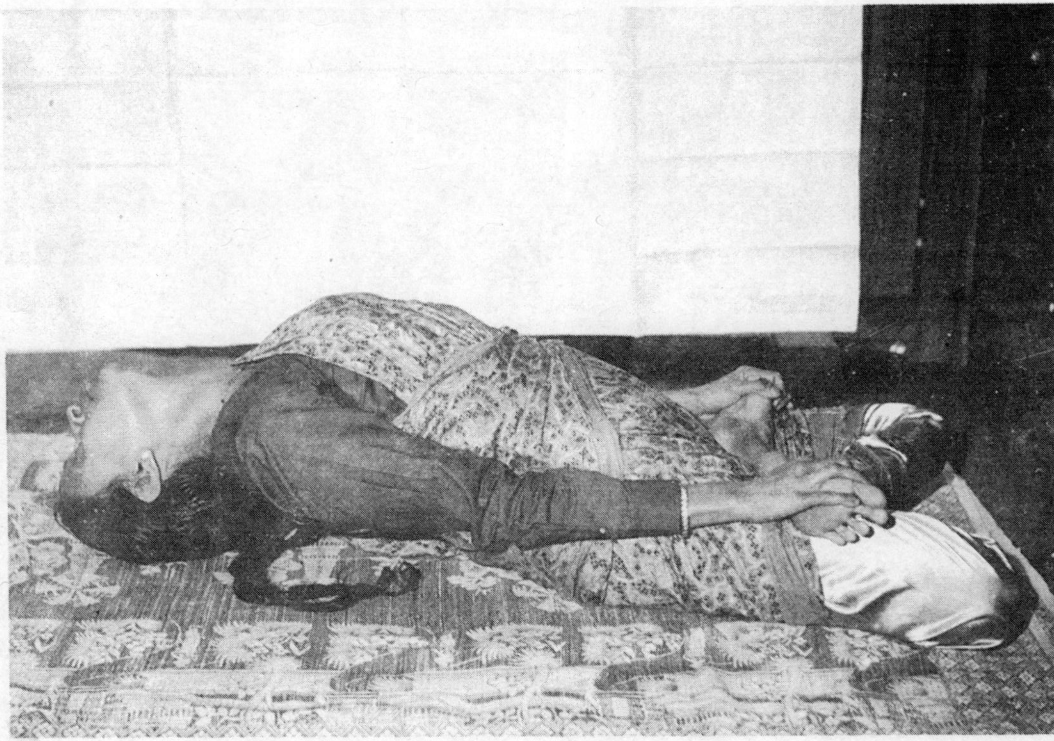

Matsyasana

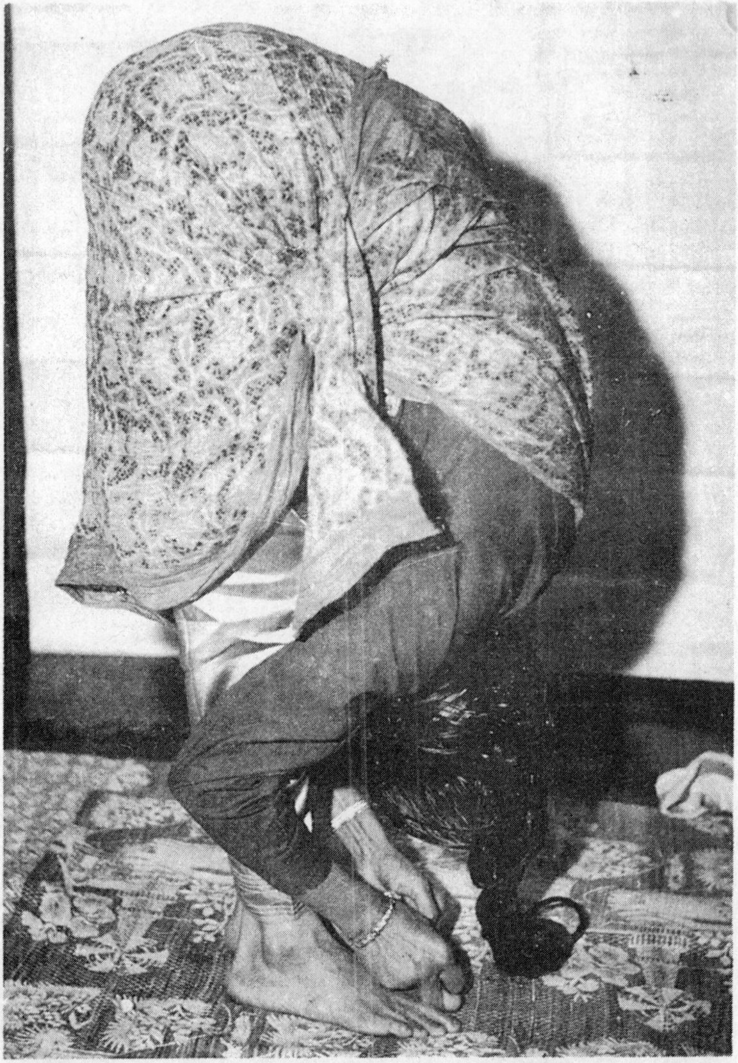

Padhahastasana

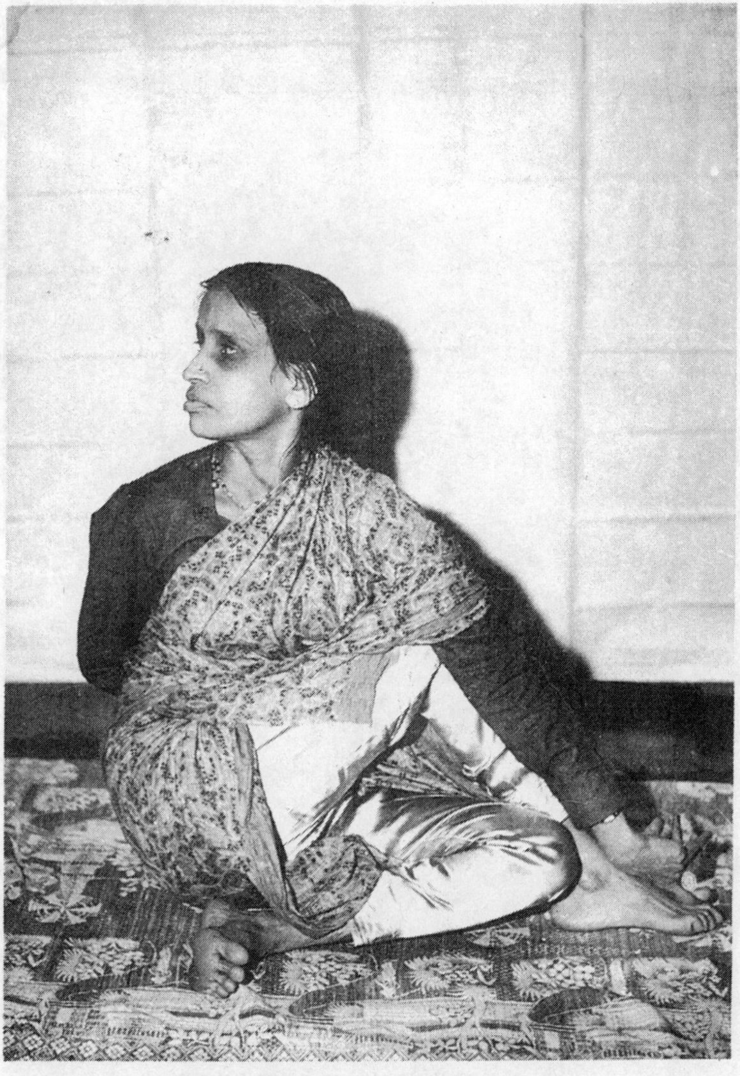

Ardha-matsyendrasana (Front-view)

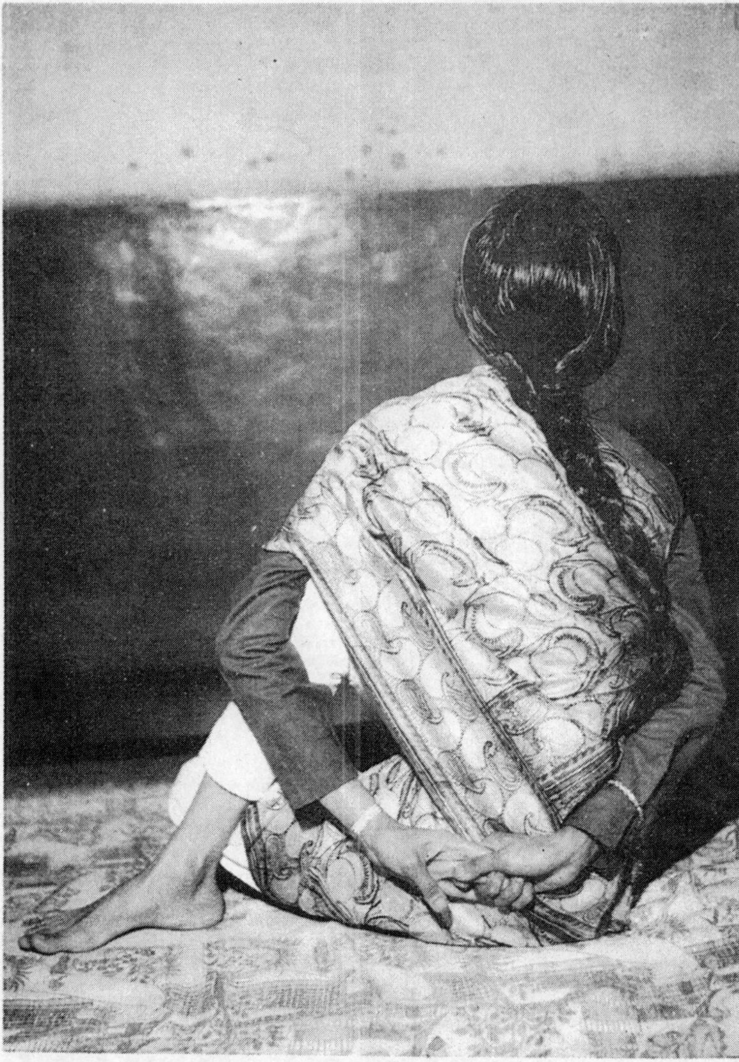

Ardha-matsyendrasana (Back-view)